A WOMAN HAS
TWICE AS MUCH FATTY TISSUE AS A MAN

When it's smoothly distributed, it gives her those appealing soft curves that are an asset to femininity. But when it gets out of control and becomes cellulite, there is twice as much area—*twice the proportion to your body's weight—where the problem can occur!* And once it does —only special measures will get rid of it!

Regular diets fail. Ordinary reducing diets can reduce your bustline to the vanishing point before even starting on the cellulite that gives hips and thighs that unsightly, lumpy look. Some diets, by putting a strain on your body, create toxic wastes that can actually increase rather than decrease the cellulite.

Do you have cellulite? Pinch yourself and see. If your skin ripples or has a lumpy texture, you have a cellulite problem. And you need this book. It reveals every secret, every technique that once cost European women a fortune, and shows how you can BANISH THOSE UNSIGHTLY CELLULITE BUMPS FOREVER.

BANISH THOSE UNSIGHTLY CELLULITE BUMPS FOREVER
was originally published by American Consumer, Inc.

Banish those unsightly cellulite bumps forever

by

Carol Ann Rinzler

PUBLISHED BY POCKET BOOKS NEW YORK

BANISH THOSE UNSIGHTLY CELLULITE
BUMPS FOREVER

American Consumer edition published 1974

POCKET BOOK edition published February, 1975

1265

contents

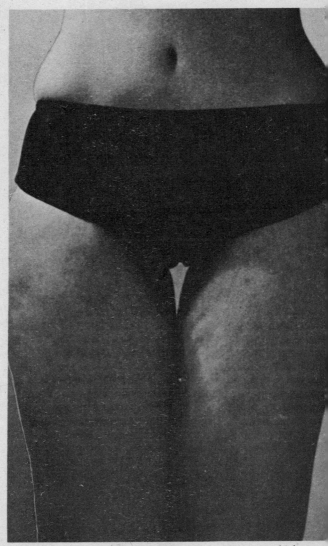

What Cellulite looks like—a moderate case on upper thighs.

Cellulite, a working definition

Cell-u-lite. **n** (cell-u-leet) The unsightly, unevenly distributed pads and lumps of fat which ordinary dieting and exercise will not dissolve. Cellulite is the legendary "last few pounds" with which serious dieters have always had to contend. It is made up of stubborn masses of fat, water and wastes which are caught in deposits at specific, vulnerable body points, such as the outer edges of the upper thighs, the hips and the knees. Trapped in the spaces just beneath the underlying fibrous network of the skin, these masses of Cellulite push against the skin's restraining fibers, bulging through the "mesh" to create the characteristic "orange peel" (or, as the French put it, **peau d'orange**) effect by which the condition may be conclusively identified.

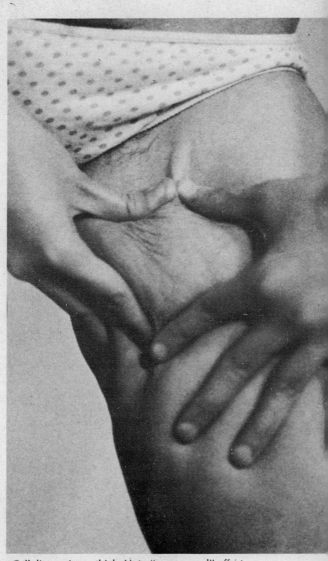

Cellulite on inner thigh. Note "orange peel" effect.

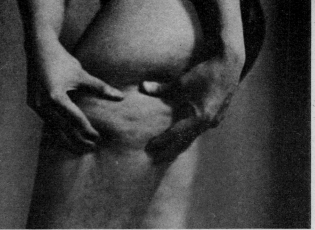
Cellulite persists, even after reducing.

(p. 10) How To Recognize the Problem

If Cellulite is present, faint dimples will appear when flesh is grasped firmly between thumb and index finger. The surface of the skin will, in fact, resemble an orange peel. In addition, affected areas may be unusually sensitive to the touch.

(p. 11) Cellulite in Advanced Stages

Skin takes on a flabby appearance. Characteristic ripples have deepened considerably and are visible without applying pressure. Large, ugly bulges develop. In most cases, increased sensitivity is no longer present.

introduction

INTRODUCTION: What is Cellulite?

Perhaps the quickest way to find out is to run your hands down the "outer edges" of your body — upper arms, hips, thighs, knees. If you find hard, bulging lumps of fat at any of these points, then you have the answer to your question.

Those hard, unsightly deposits are Cellulite, the fat which does not respond to ordinary diet and exercise programs, the traditional "last few pounds" which have always been the bedevilment of serious dieters.

Until recently, few Americans had even heard of Cellulite, although they, like their Continental cousins, had long suffered its ravages. The few who were aware that the problem had a name — and a solution — were the lucky jet-setters who had made their way to the French and Swedish spas and salons where Cellulite control was an established way of life.

Today, this program is yours for the asking. "Banish Those Unsightly Cellulite Bumps Forever" offers you the principles by which to eliminate this problem for the rest of your life. If you have the determination, the road to a smooth, Cellulite-free body is open to you. Starting right now.

part one

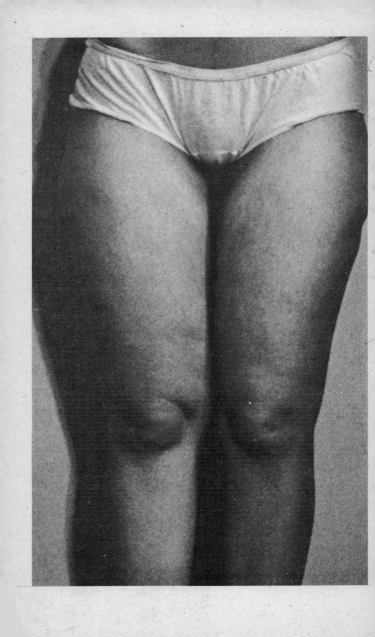

Part one: One hundred questions & answers about Cellulite control

I. The nature of the problem

1. What is Cellulite?

Cellulite is the unsightly, unevenly distributed lumps and pads of fat which ordinary dieting and exercise will not dissolve. More prosaically, it is the legendary "last few pounds" with which serious dieters have always had to wrestle.

2. How does it differ from ordinary fat?

Beneath the covering of the skin, every human being has a smooth layer of fat which serves as insulation and cushioning for the muscles and nerves. In addition, all the vital internal organs of the body are supported by small cushions of fat which protect those organs from injury. And finally, all human beings use this smooth layer of fat as a storehouse for a continuing supply of energy. This is necessary fat, and it differs from Cellulite in that it is smooth and well-distributed, a vital, functioning part of the body's essential structure. Cellulite, on the other hand, is lumpy and hard; it is found in pockets at strategic points along the body; it does not provide cushioning and insulation, nor is it the source of energy upon which the body ordinarily calls.

3. What is Cellulite made of?

Cellulite is a combination of excess fat, water and waste material which has become trapped in pockets of hard fatty substance at certain vulnerable body points.

4. What causes Cellulite?

Most Cellulite experts agree that poor diet, poor physical maintenance (the lack of an adequate exercise program) and both physical and emotional stress are the primary causes of Cellulite build-up.

5. What does it look like?

Once the Cellulite is trapped, it begins to push up against the network of holding fibers which lie just

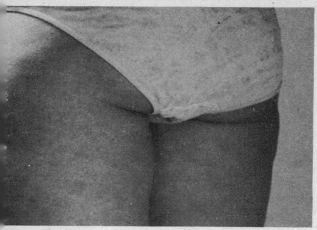

Back of thighs is another area for flabby Cellulite deposits.

beneath the skin, and bulging through the skin's restraining fibers, the Cellulite creates a characteristic "orange peel" effect, by which the condition can be conclusively identified.

6. When was Cellulite first discovered?

According to the experts, Cellulite was first identified by Swedish scientists, who created a program of massage and exercise designed to deal with it. It was popularized, however, by the French.

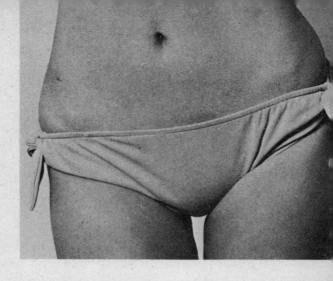

7. Why is that?

Because the French woman, with her· typically feminine figure—rounded, with flaring hips—is most likely to suffer from **coulottes de cheval,** or "riding breeches." This is a widespread form of Cellulite which consists of deposits on the upper thigh, and it is particularly inhibiting if one wishes to wear the bikinis or "strings" so popular on Continental beaches. As a result, French beauty salons had to come up with a treatment to alleviate their customers' distress, and the result was the basic Cellulite-control program which was first introduced to American readers in 1968 by **Vogue,** a magazine well known for its keen observation of the French and European beauty scenes.

8. Is Cellulite hereditary?

Obviously the tendency toward developing Cellulite is hereditary. You inherit your basic body structure from your parents, as you inherit your intelligence or the color of your hair. But that doesn't mean that you have to submit to all the possible problems that go along with your basic body type, any more than you have to settle for the color of hair you were born with. Cellulite formation can be controlled — by you.

9. Who is likely to suffer from Cellulite?

Everybody — men and women, young and old.

opposite:
Cellulite gone!

10. Are fat people more likely to have Cellulite than thin people?

Not necessarily. In fact, if you are fat enough, you may not even know you have Cellulite, since it may be layered over your body's excess fat. Only as you begin to lose weight will your Cellulite deposits become more prominently and thus more easily identified.

11. But aren't women more likely than men to have Cellulite?

No, but they are more likely to have it in prominently visible areas.

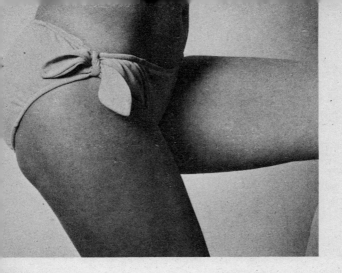

12. Why is that?

Because the sexual hormones — androgens (male) and estrogens (female) — determine both the body structure and the distribution of bodily fat. In practice, what this means is that women are more likely to find excessive fatty deposits settling on their hips and upper thighs (those **coulottes de cheval**), while in men, excessive fat is found more often on the abdomen and the upper back, around the shoulders and neck.

13. Does that mean that hormones cause fat?

Not in normal body functioning. They only determine where the fat will be.

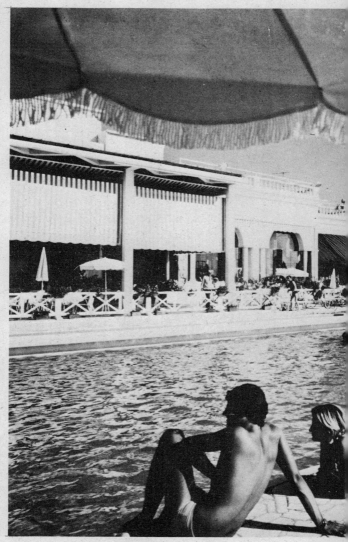

Summer is cruel

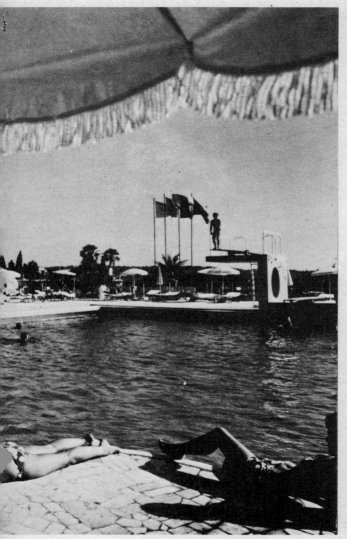

if you've got Cellulite.

14. Does my doctor know about Cellulite?

He may not, and, even if he does, he may be highly skeptical.

15. Why is that?

To begin with, **Cellulite** is not a medical term. It is a word coined by Europeans to describe a commonplace physical condition, and just because that condition — fatty deposits at strategic body points — is **so** widespread, it has been adopted as a popular designation for the condition. Any reputable doctor (and there is no other sort with whom you should deal) is right to be skeptical, cynical and downright suspicious of any popular new way to deal with weight control.

16. What is the reason for this?

There are few fields which offer as much opportunity to the quack as weight control, and, as a result, there are few fields as full of opportunity for real harm to the patient as fad diets and harmful diet regimes. Your doctor is right to protect you from such potential damage, and it is for this reason that he may look askance at a program for Cellulite control.

17. Is there an answer to his skepticism?

Yes, there is. Remember, while it is not a medical term, **Cellulite** does refer to a serious medical prob-

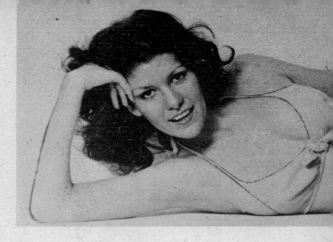

lem, the problem of ridding one's self of those fatty deposits which have heretofore evaded the serious dieter's best efforts. In addition, the Cellulite theory holds that there are two kinds of fat: The smooth, evenly distributed layer of fat which is part of the body's normal structure (and which, even when present in excess, responds steadily to sensible diet) and the lumpy, unevenly distributed fat which congregates at specific body points and resists even a motivated dieter's most conscientious attempts to dislodge it.

Knowing this, it is fascinating to discover that researchers at the Rockefeller Institute in

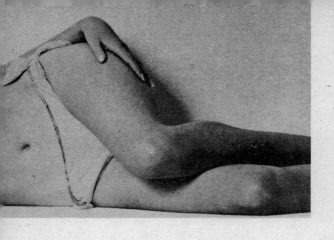

New York have evolved a theory, controversial but reputable nonetheless, which shows that fat cells in the obese differ from those in the normal individual. From this basic research Dr. Harry Gusman, who has dealt extensively with weight-control problems, has put forth his own theory, which states that there are two types of fat tissue, one normal, the other not.

The doctor says that while fat tissue is an essential part of the body, providing both structural

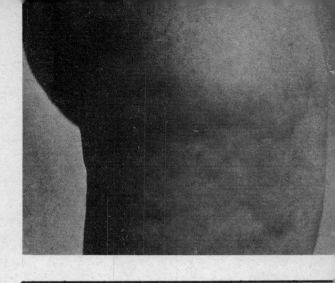

support and reserve energy, abnormal fat is **not** necessary for energy, nor is it part of the body's structure. In addition, this abnormal fat may be the precipitating factor which tips a serious dieter off his or her regime.

18. How does that happen?

The doctor explains that the dieter begins the regime severely overweight. At that point, he or she may not even be aware of the lumpy, unevenly distributed fatty deposits which lie underneath the excessive — but relatively smooth — overweight. By the time the dieter has succeeded in reducing the first layers of fat and the body is about to call upon the long-submerged reserves of the lumpy fat un-

---

derneath, he or she may well be exhausted. In addition, it is only at this point that the dieter is really aware of those ugly lumps which do not seem to be responding at all the strenuous regime to which the body has been subjected. At this point, annoyed and frustrated by the deprivation that has been endured and the apparent failure of the diet to eliminate the ugliest part of the problem, the dieter throws up his or her hands in disgust—and goes right back to eating, thus aggravating the original problem.*

19. Isn't that what Cellulite experts have been saying?

In great measure, it is.

*Neil Solomon, M.D., *The Truth About Weight Control* (New York: Dell Publishing Co., Inc.).

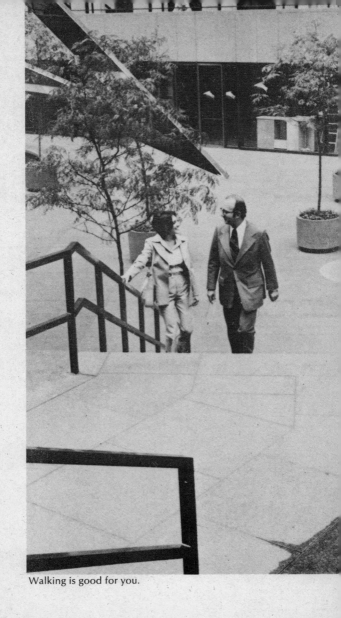
Walking is good for you.

20. What does that mean insofar as Cellulite and the medical profession are concerned?

It means that the doctors have gone about their job in the right way: Carefully, step by step. And that at the end, they have done an interesting thing, which is to validate by scientific research a popular tenet of folk wisdom.

---

21. Has this ever happened before?

Yes, it has. Digitalis and quinine, for example, are both evolved from folk medicine. (Digitalis is a product of foxglove, a plant used in English home remedies for years before doctors discovered its application to heart disease. Quinine, a product of the cinchona tree's bark, was recognized by the Andean Indians as an antifever drug long before its effectiveness against malaria was known.) And, remember when your mother used to tell you to drink a glass of milk before going to sleep? Well, Mother was right. The calcium in milk is a natural and harmless sedative, a good trick to know about instead of pills.

22. What does this mean for my Cellulite-control program?

It means that you and your doctor can work, together, as you should, to devise a serious and successful Cellulite regime. Begin with the dietary aspects of Cellulite control.

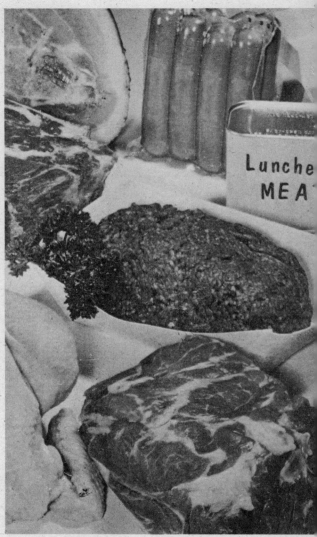

Can you spot the forbidden foods?

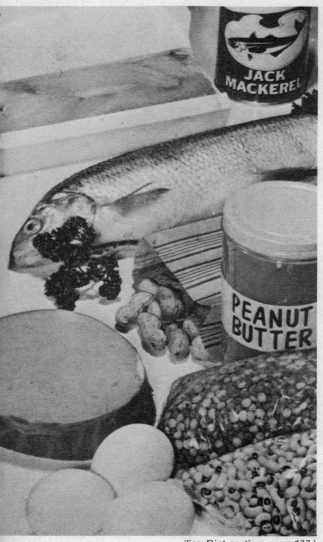

(See Diet section, page 132.)

II. Nutrition & Cellulite: Using and abusing food

23. Is diet the way to control Cellulite?

No diet alone can rid you of your ugly Cellulite deposits, for diet is only one element in your Cellulite-control program. But the proper diet can indeed be a primary factor in eliminating your present Cellulite and preventing the formation of new Cellulite.

24. I'm already on a reducing diet, and the places you describe as Cellulite-prone sound very familiar to me. Am I right?

Yes, you are. If you have been serious about your diet and your nutritional practices, you know that these places — the hips, the upper thighs, the knees — are the spots where lumps of fat still remain when you have reached almost to the end of your planned weight loss. These Cellulite pads are the "last few pounds" which are always hardest to lose.

25. If I just stick with the diet that brought me this far, won't that take care of the Cellulite?

Not necessarily. Cellulite is tricky. You probably didn't even know you had it until you were far enough along in your diet to **see** the uneven lumps

opposite:
You don't have to starve: whole wheat roll, a moderate serving of meat, green vegetables and mashed potatoes without butter, and skim milk dessert topping instead of cream.

---

and bulges of hard Cellulite. Now, the diet which took off all the previous pounds may not be the right one for removing the remaining Cellulite. In fact, it may even be working actively against you and stealthily promoting the formation of new Cellulite.

26. How?

To begin with, stress and inadequate elimination have been shown to be major causes of Cellulite formation. If your present diet is an irritating one — either because it lacks adequate calories and nutrients or because the foods you eat are themselves irritating to the body — it will produce stress within the body, contributing to the build-up of new Cellu-

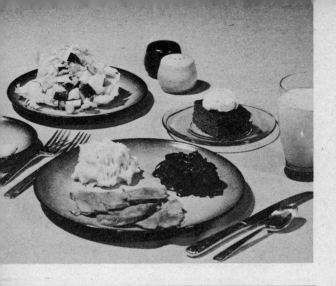

lite, rather than to the dissolution of the old. Then too, if your present diet is not geared to promoting adequate elimination of toxic waste material from your body, that, in itself, would work against you in your battle to rid yourself of Cellulite deposits.

27. How exactly would you define a diet which works against Cellulite?

Start with what it is not: It is not a diet designed to starve your body or to deprive you of the calories and nutrients you need to remain in perfect working order. It **is** a diet which will keep you at the top of your form, will eliminate stress and will promote the elimination of waste material from your body.

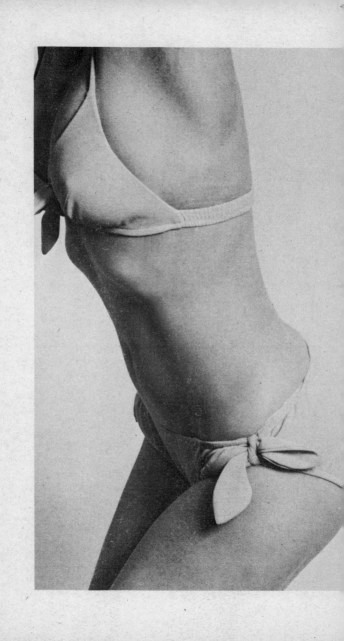

opposite:
The right diet can do this for you.

28. Is there a specific calorie count I should follow on a diet to control Cellulite?

Yes, but it varies from person to person. Dieting to control Cellulite, you should take in slightly fewer calories than you will expend in energy during the day. The amount of calories required can vary dramatically from person to person. One individual, for example, may require up to 2,500 calories during a typical day. In fact, for this individual, therefore, 2,200 calories would be a reducing diet. Another person might very well gain weight on 800 calories a day. Your personal calorie count is something you and your doctor can determine after a little experimenting. Once you know how many calories you require, you can determine exactly how many you can ingest on the Cellulite diet.

opposite:
Make sure the whole family eats right to avoid Cellulite at
all ages.

---

29. Can you give me a day-to-day diet which will work well for Cellulite?

There is a diet which, in conjunction with a well-structured program of physical maintenance, will enable you to deal successfully with Cellulite. Before we get to it, however, let's consider some of the basic principles which govern the ways in which your body uses the food you eat.

30. Is there a name for those principles?

Grouped together, they constitute the study of nutrition.

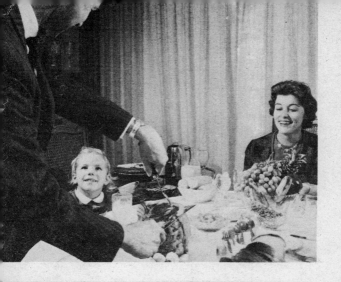

31. What does nutrition deal with?

The science of nutrition has two branches. The first deals with the processes by which your body creates tissues and energy from the foods you eat. The second deals with the number of calories and types of food your body needs to do a good job of building itself and maintaining its efficiency.

32. Exactly what does my body do with the food I eat?

It sends the food through five important steps:

First, there is the simple act of getting the food

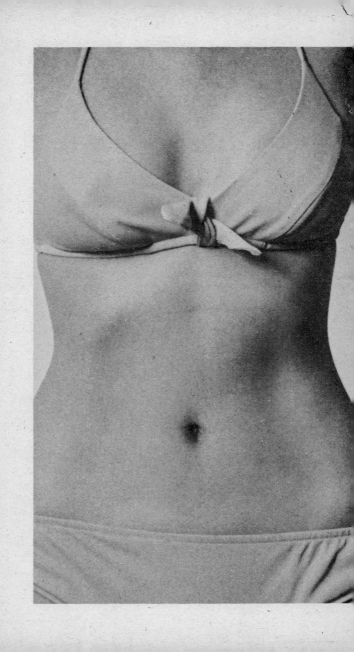

into your body, that is, taking it into your mouth, mashing it up with your teeth, and then swallowing it. Next, the food which has been sent on to your stomach is digested, which means that the enzymes in the digestive juices break it up, physically and chemically, into particles ready for the third step, absorption. Absorption is the process by which the new infinitesimal particles of food are taken from the gastrointestinal tract into your blood stream, which, in turn, speeds them into your liver for the fourth step in nutrition, assimilation. It is during assimilation that the liver transforms the food particles into materials called **amino acids,** the form in which the body can utilize them to build tissues.

opposite:
City or country, you can still get exercise.

Finally, when all the usable material has been extracted from the food you ate and turned into body tissue, your body excretes the waste matter through four major organs: The skin, the lungs, the bladder and the intestines.

33. I can understand why the body would manufacture bone, blood and muscle tissue in this process, but why does it manufacture fat, which seems so unnecessary?

As we said earlier, a certain amount of fat tissue is vital to your body's proper functioning. It serves to insulate you against drastic changes in temperature, it cushions your internal organs against shock, and it provides a means of storing energy.

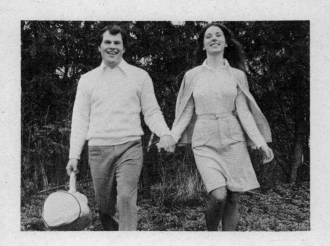

34. You mean all the energy I use comes from fat?

Not all. First you use the immediate energy available daily in the food calories you consume (that's what calories are: units of energy). Fat, however, is the best means your body has for storing up energy against a possible emergency.

35. If my body uses fat tissue as energy, why am I overweight?

When you take in more calories than you need to perform your normal activities, your fat cells, rather than excreting the excess, simply swell to take it in. Fat cells will continue to swell just as long as

---

you continue to supply them with more food. Fortunately, although most Americans do overeat, the majority of them stop feeding their fat cells long before they reach a stage of gross obesity.

36. So, simply eating too much is the reason for overweight?

It is the primary one. Although some people may suffer from metabolic disorders which only a doctor can and should identify, most overweight is produced by overeating. Scientifically, we would say that when you take in more energy sources (food) than you need to expend, the extra energy is converted into fat cells, where it is stored in anticipation

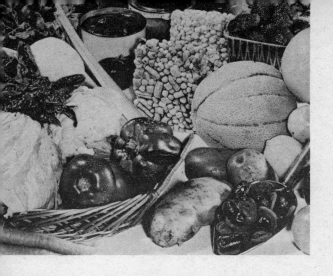

of the body's need for an emergency reserve source of fuel. Remember, your body doesn't know you aren't planning to take a 20-mile hike tomorrow, or to cut down 20 trees, or to use the energy required to solve 200 mathematics problems. All your body can do is pack away the food you feed it. If you want to change the pattern, you have the means.

37. How do I start?

You start getting after fat and Cellulite with the correct diet — again, one which will prevent stress and help in the elimination of wastes from your body.

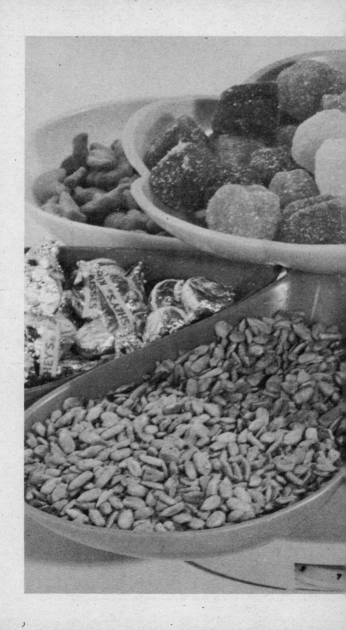

opposite:
Everything here is bad.

---

38. Are there certain foods I should avoid?

There certainly are. You should avoid all foods which are known to be irritants, pollutants, or just plain fakes.

39. Which foods are these?

Just the ones you think they are (and probably hope will not show up on the list). Spiced meats, highly fatted foods like malteds or mayonnaise, "fake" foods like potato chips and pretzels, and excessively salted foods like salted nuts. You will find a more complete list of forbidden foods in the later section on Diet.

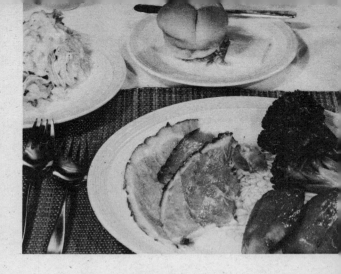

40. Are there specific foods I should include in my diet?

You should include selections from the four basic food groups—milk foods; meat, fish and fowl; vegetables and fruits; breads and cereals — in the proper proportions. Again, we will discuss the specifics when we discuss the diet for Cellulite control.

41. That sounds sensible.

It is. The essence of Cellulite control is to be sensible, to treat your body with the respect it deserves. The diet you pick — and you will have a variety from which to choose — should supply you with all the nutrients required for good health. If you have a special medical problem, your doctor is your best source for a diet tailored to your needs. But, at bottom, dieting to control Cellulite means eating sensibly so as to avoid stress and help your body cleanse itself of all irritating and polluting agents through the process of proper elimination.

42. Why is elimination important to Cellulite control?

The retention of body wastes within the tissues is a primary factor in the production of lump Cellulite fat. As a result, the elimination of these wastes, combined with a correct diet and a sensible system of physical exercise, can be of immeasurable benefit in dissolving existing Cellulite deposits and preventing the formation of new deposits.

43. How does my body cleanse itself of wastes?

Through the functioning of four major organs: The skin, the lungs, the kidneys and the intestines. We will discuss the functions of the skin and the lungs when we consider the part that exercise plays in your Cellulite-control program. Right now, let's begin with the role the kidneys play in clearing waste matter from the body.

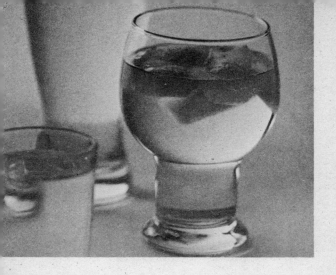

44. How do the kidneys carry wastes from the body?

The kidneys flush wastes from the body through the bladder, in the form of urine. As a result, the consumption of liquids is basic strategy in dealing with Cellulite, for the more you drink, the more efficiently your kidneys and bladder can work with you to purify the body.

45. Just any liquids?

No. There are some which are bad for you from the point of view of your kidneys as well as your Cellulite regimen.

opposite:
Skim milk is your best source of calcium.

46. What liquids should I avoid?

Two groups. The first are the irritants: Coffee, tea, alcohol, carbonated beverages. The second group are the high-caloric drinks you can do without: Malteds, ice cream sodas, very sweet synthetic drinks or "ades."

47. What liquids can I drink?

Obviously the very best drink of all is water, just plain water. And it doesn't have to be expensive imported bottled water, either. In the United States and most of Western Europe, your best bet is the inexpensive, well-cared-for water which flows right from the kitchen tap. Don't be foolish, of course, and play around with the local water when you

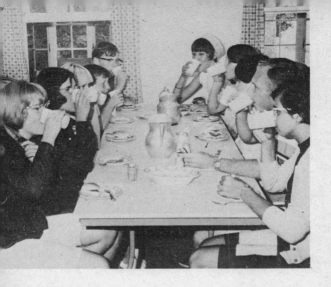

travel to areas where the sanitation isn't up to snuff, but for everyday drinking at home, go right to the kitchen tap.

48. How much should I drink each day?

The Golden Rule here is the one you learned in grammar school: six to eight glasses of water a day.

49. But, since Cellulite is composed of water, fat and wastes, won't drinking more water make more Cellulite?

Not under normal circumstances. For the most part, the idea of becoming "waterlogged" is a myth. However, there are two exceptions of which you should be aware.

---

50. What are they?

The first may occur in women as part of the normal menstrual cycle. A few days before the onset of the menstrual period, many women will experience a tendency towards bloating. It is a medical commonplace, however, that avoiding an excess of salted and spicy foods during these days can alleviate and possibly entirely do away with this problem. If bloating persists, however, a woman should consult her gynecologist.

The second exception to the rule has to do with the consumption of salt, which acts to retain water within the body tissues.

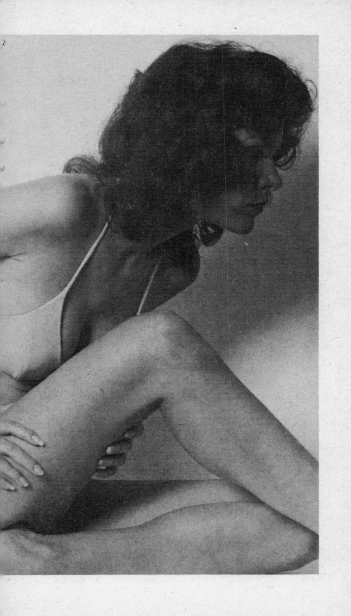

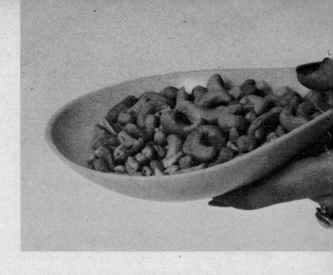

Unless you work in front of a blast furnace all day, or otherwise perspire enough to lose excessive salts from your body, you are probably consuming too much salt right now. The commonly accepted rule for dealing with this is to cut down on unnecessary, highly salted foods such as nuts, and to avoid using salt from the shaker at the table. For the normal person, these small steps should go far toward eliminating the possibility of water retention. One cautionary note, however: Before you begin to experiment with the salt balance in your diet, you should ascertain whether or not you have any problem with hypertension or heart disease. If you do, under no circumstances should you ever fiddle with the salt-controlled diet your doctor has prepared for

opposite:
Avoid temptations.

you. If you have questions, ask him. Never experiment on your own.

51. Are there any other possible adverse effects from drinking six to eight glasses of water a day?

Just one, but it is primarily a result of relying upon a fad diet. The water is an innocent accomplice.

52. What is the adverse effect?

When your kidneys are operating at peak efficiency, the urine they excrete will carry waste matter from your body. It will also carry certain substances along with the wastes. In the normal course of events, you would not miss these substances—even

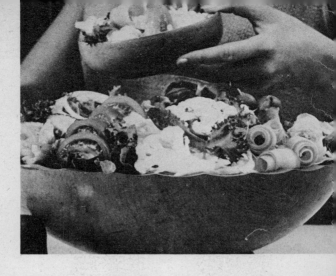

though they are necessary to your health, indeed to your life — because an adequate diet, composed of nutrients from each of the four major food groups (milk, meat, cereal, fruits/vegetables) will replenish these life-sustaining substances each day. If you confine yourself to a fad diet, however, such as one which relies upon an excessive quantity of one "magic" food to the exclusion of all others, you will be heading for serious trouble.

53. Can you give me an example?

Yes. The classic case is described by Dr. Neil Solomon in his excellent popular book on nutrition, **The Truth About Weight Control.** Dr. Solomon describes a man who, tired of continuous dieting, decided to lose weight fast, once and for all. Choosing a diet consisting of eight glasses of water a day and great quantities of lettuce, he reasoned that the bulk of the lettuce would calm his inevitable hunger pangs.

As for the water, everybody knows, he decided, that men can live for weeks at a time on water alone.

Unfortunately, he did not know how important potassium is to the body, nor did he understand that the kidneys, functioning superbly on eight glasses of water a day, would wash all the potassium right out of his system.

Deprived of replenishment, his supply of potassium dropped, and so did his blood pressure. Had his doctor not stepped in as he went into shock, his heart would have stopped as well. Such are the perils of fad dieting, and, as you can see, the water was an innocent but damaging instrument of his downfall.*

*Neil Solomon, M.D., *The Truth About Weight Control* (New York: Dell Publishing Co., Inc.).

opposite:
Pills are the lazy way, and can be dangerous.

54. Are diuretic drugs useful in fighting Cellulite?

Not really. To begin with, they are usually unnecessary. As you have learned, unless you are using too much salt, or are pre-menstrual, or are suffering from a serious medical problem which would require your doctor's intervention, your Cellulite-control program of diet and physical maintenance will enable your healthy body to excrete excess water and body wastes through normal urination. For this reason, most doctors will advise against the use of diuretic drugs unless there is obvious disease which requires them. (In this regard, it should be one of your own iron-clad health rules never to prescribe such drugs for yourself, or to "borrow" a friend's — only your doctor should prescribe medicine.) If your

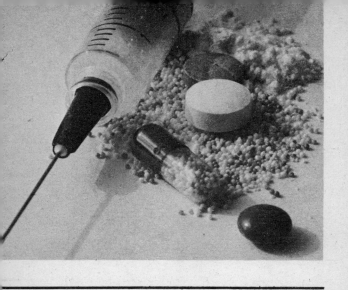

doctor agrees, you can, however, use the mild, natural diuretics, called **tisanes,** or teas, which you can brew from various herbs, fruits or vegetables. Try your local health store for ideas. The delicious scents alone are worth the trip.

55. Then those six to eight glasses of water a day will do the trick?
Yes.

56. What is the function of the intestines in Cellulite control?
Just as the kidneys and bladder work to purify the body by eliminating wastes through urination, the intestines function to eliminate solid wastes.

57. How important is "regularity"?

It is important that your body rid itself of its solid wastes, but so long as your digestive processes are working properly, the frequency with which this occurs can vary widely from person to person. It depends upon a number of factors — your age, the amount of exercise you perform, the kind of food you eat, the amount of food you eat, and, at times, your emotional state of mind. Doctors report that "normal" regularity can vary from two bowel movements a day to two a week.

58. Why do I become constipated when I start on a new diet?

There are three probable reasons: The first is

that your new diet probably has less fat than you are accustomed to consuming, so that there is less lubrication in the bowels. In addition, you are now eating less food, which would certainly result in a lesser amount of solid waste to be eliminated. Finally, most people drink less when they first start a new diet, and this, too, can cause constipation.

59. Should I use laxative drugs?

Never without your doctor's consent. Like diuretic drugs, laxatives are usually unnecessary and may often be harmful. It is far more healthful to rely upon the natural laxatives which are so important a part of your Cellulite-control program.

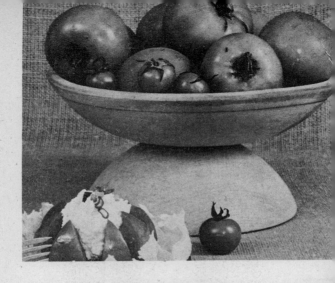

60. What are they?

Proper diet, regular exercise and the same six to eight glasses of water which we discussed earlier.

61. How do they work?

The proper diet will provide the essential "bulk" foods: Raw fruits and vegetables. When calories are not an overriding concern, prunes are the natural laxative, **par excellence.** Regular exercise will strengthen the muscles of your stomach and digestive tract, just as it affects all the other muscles in your body, and an adequate supply of liquids is just as important to the elimination of solid wastes as it is to the elimination of wastes through the kidneys and bladder, for it helps to ease the passage of solid, dry waste material through the intestines.

62. If I eat right and keep my body in working order, will I be able to control my Cellulite problem?

Yes, provided you combine good diet with the good exercise hints which you find in the next chapter. Remember, neither diet alone, nor exercise alone will eliminate Cellulite — the real answer is a combination of both which adds up to a complete Cellulite-control program.

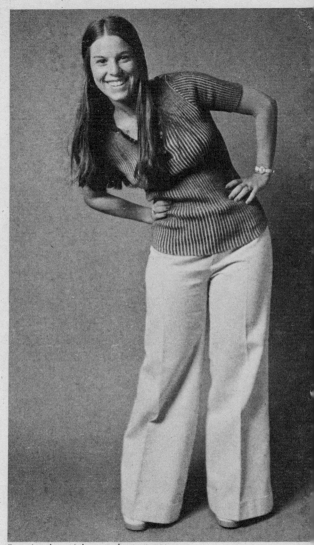
Exercise doesn't have to be torture.

III. Exercise: The Value of Physical Maintenance

63. What is the role of exercise in my Cellulite-control program?

Along with a proper diet, a well-planned exercise program will help your body to dissolve existing Cellulite deposits and prevent the formation of new ones.

64. How?

Sensible exercising promotes a sensation of all-over well-being which can go far towards alleviating the stresses of everyday life which have been shown to be a major factor in Cellulite formation. Most important, correct exercise assists your body in eliminating the waste material which would otherwise contribute to the maintenance or proliferation of those ugly lumps and bulges.

opposite:
The benefits are beautiful.

65. Shouldn't exercise also "burn off" fat?

If you expend more energy than you take in, that is, if you eat less and exercise more, your body will begin to call upon the excess energy which is stored in the layer of fat which covers your structure. The use of this stored energy will indeed "burn off" fat. However, by the time you get to Cellulite, the "last few pounds" which have defied the best efforts of your regular diet, most of the excess fat has already disappeared. What remains is Cellulite, and, since excess waste material is a major cause of Cellulite, the primary aim of your exercising — just as it is the primary aim of your diet — is to eliminate wastes from the body.

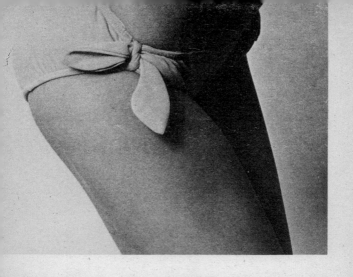

66. How does exercise do this?

By promoting the efficient operation of the skin and lungs, two of the four major organs of elimination (the kidneys and the intestines are the other two).

67. How does exercise help the skin eliminate waste?

Although the skin, like the lungs, is an organ of respiration, its major excretory function is performed through perspiration. Perspiration is a highly efficient way of removing wastes from the body. (As a matter of fact, it may sometimes be **too** efficient,

opposite:
Salt tablets: don't use them without your doctor's advice.

which is why persons who constantly engage in activities which promote an abundance of perspiration are often advised by their doctors to use salt tablets to replenish the quantities of salt which are excreted from the body. People involved in normal activities, however, will not lose salt to that extent.)

68. Doesn't perspiration also result in a quick loss of weight?
    If it is copious enough, it will, but the loss will be only temporary, at best.

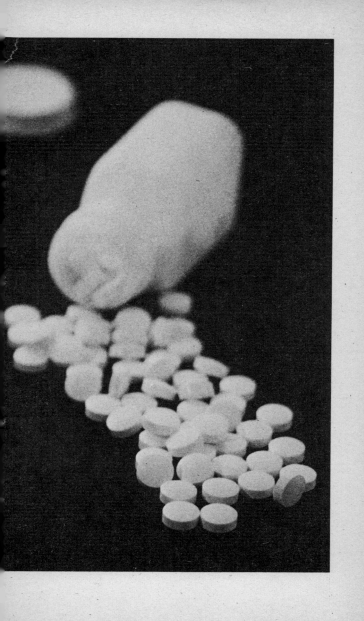

69. Why?

Because it is a loss of "water weight" only, and the healthy body will — and should — replace it. However, the loss is often so dramatic that "crash" dieters regard sauna baths and other perspiration-inducing activities as miraculous aids to reducing. If you are serious about getting rid of Cellulite, you would do best to ignore the "miracles" and concentrate on the purifying aspects of perspiration.

70. Does the skin eliminate wastes in any other ways?

Like the lungs, the skin is also an organ of respiration. It can bring oxygen into the body and release

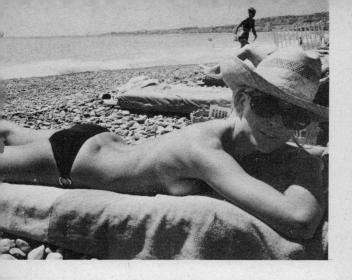

wastes through the pores. That is one reason why many health experts advocate "skin baths," that is, nude relaxation or exercise.

71. What effect does exercise have on the lungs?

Properly performed, it increases their capacity to supply oxygen to the various organs of the body.

72. Why is that important?

In order for your body to perform even the simplest task, it must convert food into energy, and oxygen is the essential fuel which allows this conversion to take place. In addition, oxygen is required to rid the body of various by-products of energy-conversion, namely carbon dioxide. Without sufficient oxygen, therefore, there can be serious complications.

73. What are they?

For one thing, carbon dioxide will begin to build up, and, as a result, everything will slow down. Your brain won't think quickly, your muscles won't work right, and your entire body will feel heavy and "logy." If you live in an area which has periods of heavy smog, you have already experienced this feeling on days when air pollution reduces your oxygen supply.

A second complication is that the lack of oxygen

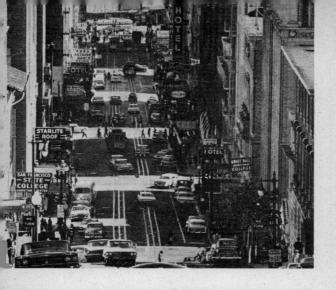

can increase the possibility of blood-clotting, which is why cardiologists usually recommend a sensible program of exercise for patients with heart disease. In sum, both exercise and proper breathing are essential to the elimination of waste from the body, a concern which is central to your Cellulite-control program.

74. How do I go about getting more oxygen into my lungs?

Start with that old standby which you learned in grammar school along with the Golden Rule about drinking six to eight glasses of water a day: Stand up straight. Good posture is more than a simple exercise for children. It is the only position in which

opposite:
Stand up straight . . . but don't exaggerate.

---

your body will allow your lungs the maximum
amount of room in which to expand within the rib
cage during inspiration, or breathing-in. Take a look
at the difference yourself. Stand in front of your bedroom mirror and hunch yourself over so that your
chest bends in towards your stomach and your
entire body forms an uncomfortable, constricted
C-curve. Your lungs can't possibly do their job in
that position, and if they can't do their job of bringing the oxygen in, you are going to be mighty uncomfortable.

75. How can I correct this?

As we said, you start by standing up straight. You
don't have to walk around like a West Point cadet

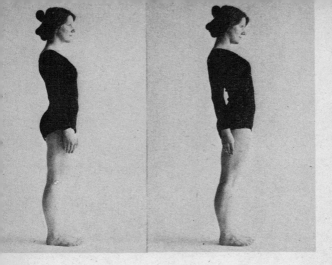

with your chin tucked in to your chest. As a matter of fact, this artifically straight pose can be just as detrimental to good breathing as that messy old C-curve. What you have to do is simply counteract your normal desire to bend your neck, lower your head, and generally assume the aspect of an untidy piece of spaghetti.

76. Wait a minute. Did you say that was normal?

Sure. If man were back on all fours where he started, the curved-down head would be a normal position. Standing up on two legs, you find that your torso is a heavy burden for your legs and your head and neck are an even heavier burden for your spine. Nobody argues the fact that it's hard to stand up straight, but the truth is that once you get the hang of it, it is much less fatiguing in reality than your old hang-dog posture **seemed** to be.

77. Once I'm standing up straight, what do I do?

Breathe. Pull the air into your lungs and be certain to expand your diaphragm as you do. Many children, back in that old grammar school, were told that it was necessary to pull in their stomachs (really their diaphragms) when they breathed. This is physical nonsense. Your aim is to fill your lungs up with air, and a pulled-in diaphragm will keep your lungs from expanding as much as possible. Once

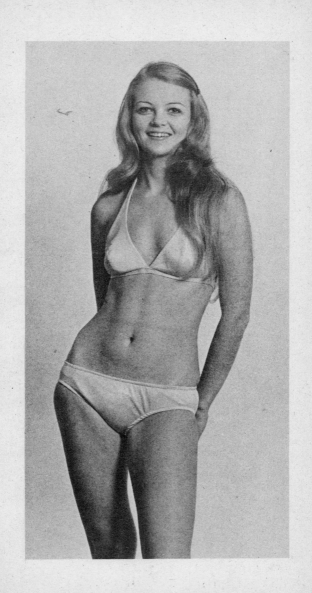

you've got the air in, let it out. You'll be sending out lots of unnecessary carbon dioxide along with it.

78. Is it really that simple?

Yes, it is, but doing it the right way will make a truly astonishing difference in your ability to move with vigor and to think decisively. In addition, you will be cutting down drastically on the accumulation of the waste material which is a primary cause of Cellulite formation and retention.

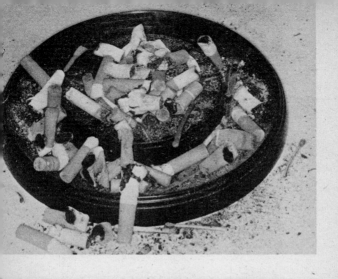

79. While we're on the subject of breathing, what about cigarettes and Cellulite?

It's hard to think of anything good to say about cigarettes in ordinary circumstances, but when it comes to the question of Cellulite control, it's downright impossible. Remember, those ugly Cellulite deposits are a result of wastes which build up within the body, and smoking is probably the worst body-polluter of them all. It brings foreign substances into the body through the lungs and bloodstream; it cuts down on the body's ability to get oxygen and contributes to the build-up of carbon dioxide; it slows the process of digestion and elimination; it speeds up the heart beat; and recent studies have even shown that smokers have more facial wrinkles than

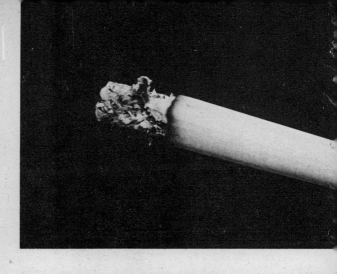

non-smokers. Surely the temporary, though acute, discomfort of withdrawal from cigarettes is worth the long-term benefits. And, interestingly enough, the increased water consumption and regular exercise of your Cellulite-control program, may help to alleviate the symptoms which accompany quitting.

80. Once I give up smoking, which exercises will work best to combat Cellulite?

Those which increase the oxygen in your system; those which produce an all-over "smoothing" effect; and those which go directly to work on a specific problem area — hips, thighs, upper arms, and so forth.

opposite:
That's carbon monoxide, right to your lungs.

---

81. Which exercises bring in more oxygen?

Those which require an intensive, all-out effort. Jumping rope is a fine example. As a matter of fact, it's such a terrific, all-around exercise that there's a whole book, **Jump for Joy,*** devoted to its many variations. The old-fashioned warm-up exercise, the Jumping Jack—you'll find a picture and description of this, along with other Cellulite-control exercises, in the section on "Your Personal Cellulite Control Program"—is another good example.

82. What about running in place—doesn't that meet the standards?

No. Unlike jumping rope and the Jumping Jack, running in place puts more stress on some muscles than others and is likely to produce muscle bulges to compete with your Cellulite bumps.

*Roy Ald, *Jump for Joy* (New York: Bernard Geis Assoc., Inc.).

opposite:
This is not the way to exercise.

83. Which exercises have an all-over "smoothing" effect?

Walking, swimming and modern dance. Unlike the more "athletic" pursuits, such as tennis, ballet or horseback riding, these will promote the smooth, even distribution of flesh which is your eventual goal. In addition, these are exercises you can move into gradually and practice on a more or less daily basis. You can walk to work or to your daily errands; you can perform the movements of modern dance in the privacy of your own living room or bedroom; and you can swim at the local pool, beach or health club.

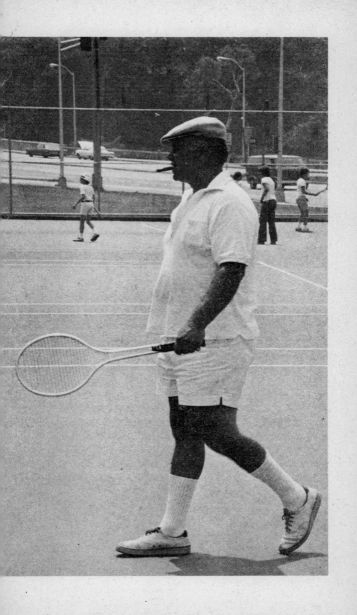

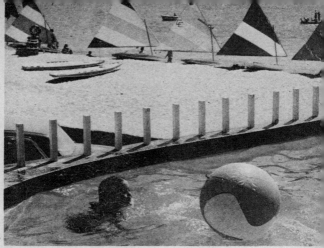

This is better . . .

84. How does "spot reducing" (specific exercises for specific areas) work to break up Cellulite?

By promoting increased circulation within the muscles which cover the affected area, thus speeding up the elimination of waste material from that part of the body. Keeping the muscles in working order, moreover, will lessen the chances of accumulating future Cellulite deposits.

85. Will exercise machines give the same results?

Not unless **you** do the exercise. For example, a "bicycle machine" which requires that you perform the bicycling motions will help to cut down deposits over the thighs and hips. (At the same time, however, it may contribute to bulging muscles in the

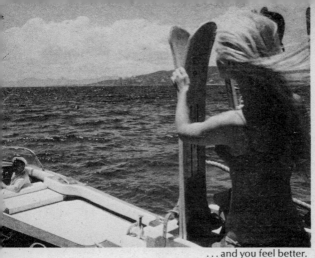

... and you feel better.

calves.) A machine which sprays warm water or warm air isn't really going to do anything but relax you, which is an admirable accomplishment, but hardly has the efficiency of a correctly maintained exercise plan. Finally, since most of these machines simply perform a kind of automated massage, why not pass them by and do the massage yourself? That way you get the benefit of a soothing massage, plus the physical activity of performing it yourself.

86. How long should I exercise each day?

You should walk — or swim, if you can — at least an hour a day. If you choose walking, this will fit easily into your daily routine. As for the oxygenating and "spot reducing" exercises, you should start with

opposite:
What a wonderful way to relax.

---

10 minutes and work up to no more than 25. Remember, your object is to make yourself smooth and healthy, not to work yourself into exhaustion.

87. Will massage break up Cellulite?

Most exercise experts say, yes; most medical men say, no; but their disagreement may be more apparent than real. What the medical men object to is terminology which suggests that massage will "break up" fatty Cellulite deposits and melt them away like so much butter. The truth is that massage can promote better circulation within the affected area, thereby promoting the increased elimination of waste material.

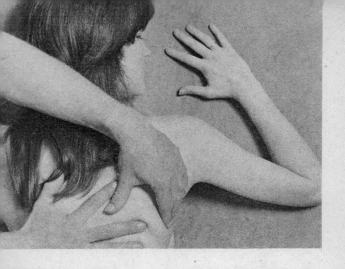

88. Are there other benefits to massage?

Yes. Massage can promote perspiration, which helps your skin to eliminate wastes. It can improve skin tone, and it can be superbly relaxing, leaving you ready to face the problems of the day with the serenity which comes from knowing that your body feels good and acts well.

89. How important is this feeling of serenity?

Very. By now you know that stress contributes to the formation of Cellulite. Caught in a stressful situation, you may not eat properly, and when you do eat, your tension will interfere with your digestive processes. In addition, your rate of breathing may quicken and become shallower, depriving you of

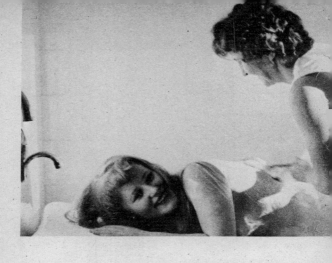

needed oxygen; and, as a result, your body will step up its production of waste material, such as carbon dioxide. At the same time, all your organs of elimination — skin, lungs, kidneys and intestines — will perform inefficiently, if at all — and there you are, caught in a Cellulite-producing cycle. Sensible massage seeks to prevent this.

90. Can massage ever be harmful?

Only if you overdo. No massage should ever leave you with serious aches and pains, or, worse, black and blue. Avoid like the plague any masseuse or technique which produces these results. Aside from the obvious point that no voluntary treatment should leave you with injuries, there is the basic fact

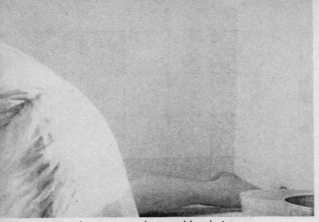
Professional massage can be superbly relaxing.

that too much such pressure can produce more Cellulite.

91. How?

By creating the very stress you seek to avoid, the same stress which should warn you away from too-rigorous dieting or over-exhausting exercise. Cellulite production is increased, not slowed, by the stress which occurs when your Cellulite deposits are traumatized or insulted.

92. Is self-massage better than a massage at the hands of a professional masseuse?

Both offer positive benefits: Massage performed by a professional has the advantage of offering you

---

complete relaxation; self-massage has the advantage of working more than one set of muscles at a time. In addition, once you have mastered the art of self-massage, you can incorporate it into your daily Cellulite-control program, performing it at your own convenience.

93. How can I learn the techniques?

You will find them described in the section on "Your Personal Cellulite Control Program" which follows, although the fact is, you probably know a great deal about them already.

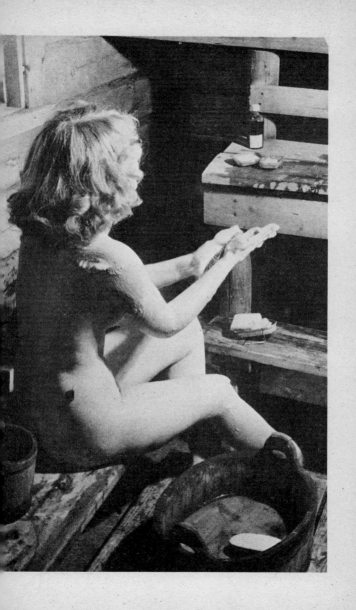

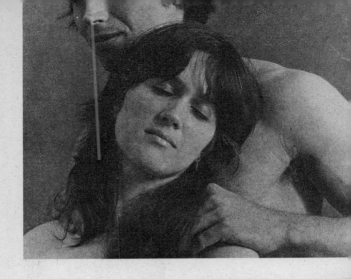

94. What do you mean?

Remember the last time you had a headache, and you reached back to rub the muscles of your upper neck? Or, when you took a shower this morning and rubbed the soap around your body? Or, when you rub, or massage, cream into your arms and legs? Have you noticed how you seem almost naturally to fall into a specific rhythm? That's massage in its most basic form.

95. Surely a Cellulite-control program of massage is more formal than that?

Of course, but the basics are as simple as the things you do every day. Remember, the aim of the

opposite:
. . . And it's even more fun together.

Cellulite-control program is to stick to basics which can be followed easily so that Cellulite control becomes second nature.

96. Can I make massage a part of my daily routine?

As we said, the best thing about self-massage is that it can be accomplished almost anywhere at any time you choose. While it might be ideal to perform the massage right before bed or after your bath, there is no reason why you can't reach down to massage your upper thigh while you are sitting in the office or at a concert, and no one will notice if you massage your upper arm while you are waiting for

opposite:
Rough towels stimulate circulation.

your lunch order to be served. Just don't make a fuss about it. Your aim is massage, not attention.

97. I've heard that there's a special cream which helps break down fatty deposits if you massage it into the skin. Is that true?

Creams can make your skin soft and supple, but none of them can penetrate to dissolve your Cellulite deposits by chemical action.

98. Well, are there any tools which can help make my massage more effective?

Yes; a simple, rough terry cloth towel or a **loofah** (a kind of rough fabric mitt or strap which is popular

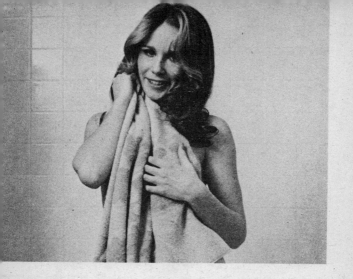

in Europe) can promote skin circulation, increasing the flow of blood to the Cellulite areas, thus increasing the elimination of wastes. A good, stiff bath brush can perform the same function, and as a bonus, these treatments will slough off the rough, dead cells of your skin's outer layer, leaving you as soft and silky as a baby.

99. Is bathing of help in getting rid of Cellulite?

Only if, as we have discussed, it promotes perspiration. On the other hand, bathing and showering can — each in different ways — provide a feeling of utter relaxation, which is always beneficial.

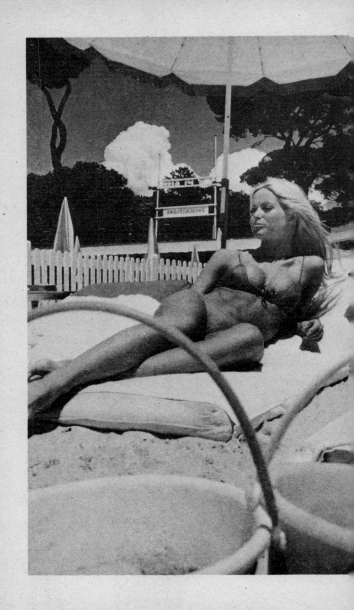

opposite:
Diet, exercise, massage—together they make a new you.

---

100. Is that the last element in my Cellulite-control program?

Yes. The proper diet — one which will cleanse your body of excess wastes — combined with a physical maintenance program which will assist in the elimination of waste while keeping you in top physical form, these are the elements which can make Cellulite control a reality. Now, it's up to you.

part two

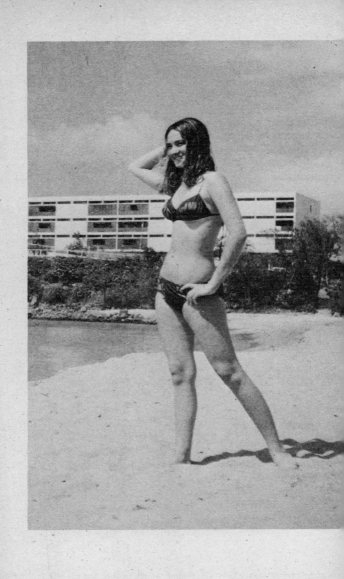

Part two: your personal cellulite control program

Your Cellulite Notebook

The key to success in your battle against the ugly ravages of Cellulite is just one word: Caring. If you care enough to follow the requirements of the Cellulite diet and exercise program, if you care enough to learn the simple, but effective, massage techniques which can banish Cellulite from your body forever — then you can win your battle.

And make no mistake, it is worth the caring. Looking well and feeling well are your rights as an attractive human being. Looking better, you will face each day with enthusiasm and with energy for the tasks which lie ahead of you. Feeling better, knowing that your body is in tune with itself, that you are no longer carrying around an ugly burden of extra flab and fat, you will have the psychological and physical

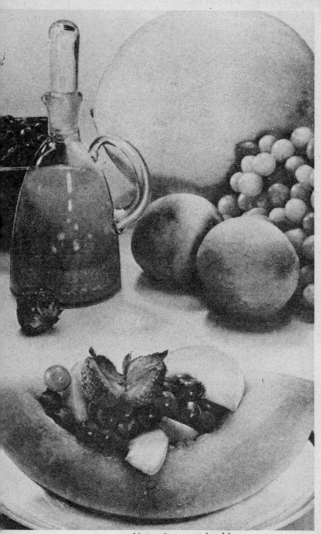
Nature's way to health.

opposite:
You're on your way.

wherewithal to become the very best that it is possible for you to be.

Once you have established the worth of the program upon which you are about to embark, you will
be ready to draw up a plan which suits you best, to
personalize the Cellulite diet and physical maintenance regimen so that it is designed specifically to
meet your Cellulite problems. (Most people do not
have to cope with the entire range of possible Cellulite defects, since the majority of us, whether
through heredity or because of previous poor diet
and exercise, have certain definite body areas which
are crying out for attention.)

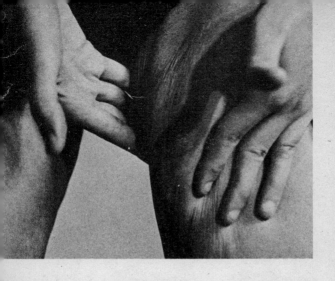

Your diet should reflect your personal prefer-
ences, for this will make it most effective for you.
While it is vital to include foods from the four major
food groups — meat, milk products, cereals, fruits
and vegetables — in every day's meal schedule,
there is no reason why you can't shift around to
your favorites, so long as you maintain a variety.

Once again, the Cellulite-control program aims to
be sensible and, insofar as is possible, convenient
enough so that it can become a habitual part of your
life.

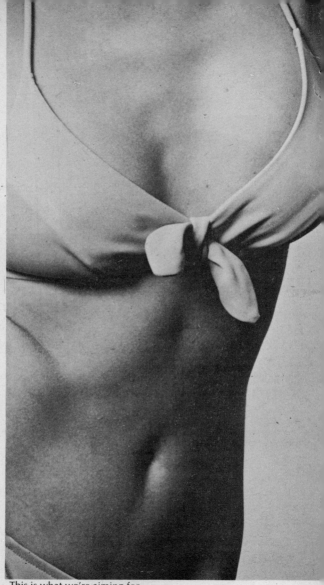

This is what we're aiming for.

The First Step

Your personal Cellulite-control program should start with a little exercise, a short walk to your stationery store, where you are going to purchase the notebook in which you will construct and record your personal regime. The best sort of notebook for this is a standard one, the small looseleaf binder which comes with a packet of ruled paper. In addition, you may wish to purchase some adhesive tabs with which to divide the notebook into various sections.

Section #1

Area	Pro- posed loss/ inches	Week #1	Week #2	Wee #:
Upper arm				
Midriff				
Waist				
Hips				
Thighs				
Knees				

The first section in your Cellulite notebook should clearly state the goals you are setting for yourself. One good way to do this is to set up a mercilessly accurate record of your body measurements. Don't

ctual Measurements

Week #4	Week #5	Week #6	Week #7	Week #8

shrink from being accurate; remember, those bulging pockets on your thighs and hips will be responding to the Cellulite diet and exercises. In a few weeks, everything will look much better.

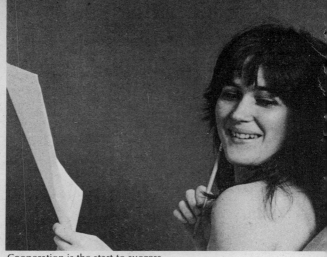

Cooperation is the start to success.

Record your measurements once a week. Try to pick the same day, and the same time of day, for this weekly ritual, as this will give you the most accurate picture of a changing body structure.

You should also keep a record of your weight, so that you will have ample warning of any sudden gain, a development which will lead you to cut down slightly on your daily calorie intake.

Do not be over-zealous in this. Undereating is as bad for Cellulite control as overeating, for both

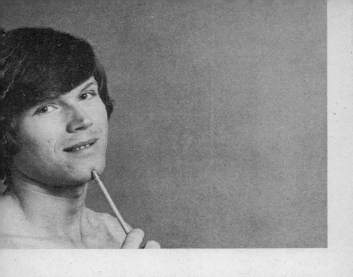

cause stress. In addition, it is neither necessary — nor, in most cases, possible—to be as flat as a board.

Instead, just pick the weight at which you perform most comfortably and efficiently, and aim to stay within three pounds of that.

Remember: Your primary aim is to rid yourself of unsightly, uneven Cellulite bumps and bulges, while maintaining your body within a state of good nutritional and physical health. Starvation diets are **out.**

Proposed ideal weight:	
Actual weight:	
Week #1	
Week #2	
Week #3	
Week #4	
Week #5	
Week #6	
Week #7	
Week #8	

Section #2

Your weekly shopping list is a major weapon in the war against Cellulite. By planning a week's menus in advance and then buying only those items which are necessary for the preparation of the meals you have selected, you can avoid the impulse buying which wastes money and clutters your kitchen shelf with irritating, polluting, fake and fattening foods.

You should jot down items daily. Each time you run out of a staple, note it down. When you want to cook something special, note it down. And remember, it isn't necessary to be fanatic in the meals and foods you plan. By the time you are into the swing of your Cellulite-control program you will know by instinct which of the foods from the four major food groups should appear in your daily fare, and, eventually, you will begin to shop with a sure knowledge of what works for you.

Section #3

Just as a doctor must read dozens of journals each month in order to keep up with medical developments, so you should read as many magazines, books and newspapers as possible in an effort to learn what new techniques and exercises are available to help in your battle against Cellulite.

This section of your personal Cellulite notebook should provide a page apiece for each new solution for one of your body's problem areas.

New developments in exercise or massage which can affect each area should be listed, along with the source from which they come, so that you can return to check the original, if that is necessary.

You will probably be finding these new techniques at an increasing rate in the next few years, for, as Cellulite control becomes better known in this country, new information will begin to flood the various magazines and newspapers. You owe it to yourself to be as well-informed as possible, in effect, to create a personalized Cellulite "encyclopedia," a collection of information which works best for you.

Area:

_____

_____

_____

_____

_____

Exercise/massage:

_____

_____

_____

_____

_____

Source (magazine, newspaper, book, salon):

_____

_____

_____

_____

_____

Results:

_____

_____

_____

_____

_____

Area:

_____
_____
_____
_____
_____

Exercise/massage:

_____
_____
_____
_____
_____

Source (magazine, newspaper, book, salon):

_____
_____
_____
_____
_____

Results:

_____
_____
_____
_____
_____

Area:

_____
_____
_____
_____
_____

Exercise/massage:

_____
_____
_____
_____
_____

**Source (magazine, newspaper,
   book, salon):**

_____
_____
_____
_____
_____

Results:

_____
_____
_____
_____
_____

Area:

_____
_____
_____
_____
_____

Exercise/massage:

_____
_____
_____
_____
_____

Source (magazine, newspaper, book, salon):

_____
_____
_____
_____
_____

Results:

_____
_____
_____
_____
_____

opposite:
The whole family can enjoy the Cellulite-control regime.

Section #4

Finally, your Cellulite notebook should end with a collection of quick-help, first-aid telephone numbers: A listing of the people who help keep you in shape.

That means:

☐ Your doctor (and an emergency number of the county medical association or other local service which can provide a doctor when yours is not available).

☐ Your masseuse (for those times when you need a professional, soothing hand to complement your self-massage program).

☐ Your gym or health club (for the swimming pool

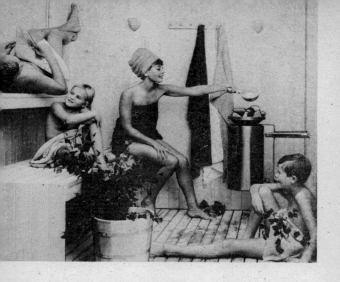

or sauna bath you do not have at home, as well as for occasional companionship in an exercise program).

☐ Your beauty salon (for that invaluable lift on days when you can't face another step of exercise, or, more happily, to make the most of the new, Cellulite-free You).

And that's it. Your Cellulite notebook isn't magic, but it can be an invaluable aid by helping you to formalize your Cellulite-control program, and make it an integral part of your daily life. Use the notebook well and regularly, and it will return benefits many times over.

The Cellulite Control Diet

The Cellulite-control diet is not a reducing regimen. Rather, it is a **cleansing** diet, designed to help your body rid itself of the noxious wastes and pollutants which are a primary cause of Cellulite formation.

Because it relies upon sound nutritional principles and includes selections from each of the four major food groups — meat, milk, grain, and fruits/vegetables — the Cellulite-control diet is compatible with any other healthful diet. It may be tailored to your personal needs simply by eliminating the specific foods which your doctor has advised you to avoid (to be certain, always check with your physician before starting any new dietary regime).

Finally, the foods on the Cellulite-control diet are widely available, making this a diet which you can follow easily in a variety of circumstances. You won't need special — and often inaccessible — preparations; just your own intelligence and the will to work your way to Cellulite control.

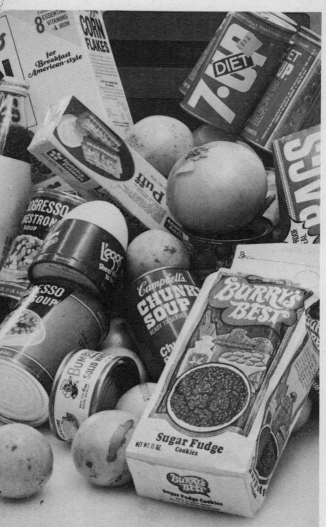

A typical checkout counter—but you're allowed only the corn flakes, onions and oranges.

Meat,
Fish,
Poultry

The prescribed methods for cooking foods in this group are broiling, baking, and roasting, all of which can produce delicious fare. But don't ignore the intrinsic value of a fine stew. Not only is it tasty, but it offers you the opportunity to combine several foods in one satisfying dish, thus saving time and energy in the preparation. Just be certain you follow two simple rules — use only water or tomato juice as your stewing liquid (in the case of fish, you may substitute clam juice), and be certain to let the stew cool before you serve it, so that you can remove the hardened fat from the top.

You
May Eat:

Veal
Lean beef (three times per week)
Chicken (without skin)
Turkey (without skin)
Organ meat (heart, liver)*
Lean fish (sole, flounder)
Shellfish (shrimp, lobster,
oysters, clams)*
Canned fish (in water or
tomato sauce, only)

*Persons on low-cholesterol diets should check with their physicians before including shellfish or organ meat in their diets.

You May Not Eat:

Spiced luncheon meats
Sausages (frankfurters,
   liverwurst, bologna,
   etc.)
Smoked meats
Smoked fish
Canned fish (in oil)
Pork
Bacon
Ham
Duck
Lamb
Goose
Thick or spicy gravies and
   sauces

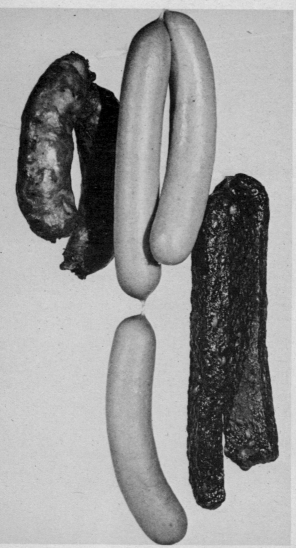

Absolutely forbidden!

Milk and
Milk Foods

Milk provides the calcium that keeps your bones and teeth healthy, and should be a part of your everyday diet after childhood is past. Adults, however, can take their milk in a variety of forms, such as those listed below.

You
May Eat:

Skim milk
Skim milk yoghurt*
Skim milk cheeses (cottage cheese,
farmer cheese, ricotta)
Hard cheeses (cheddar, American
cheddar, Jarlsberg) in moderation
Ice milk
Corn, peanut, or soybean oil margarines
instead of butter

*Frozen yoghurt makes a delicious substitute for ice cream.

You May Not Eat:

Regular Milk
Buttermilk
Butter
Sweet cream
Sour cream
Processed cheeses
"Soft" cheese (cream
cheese, Boursin,
Camembert)

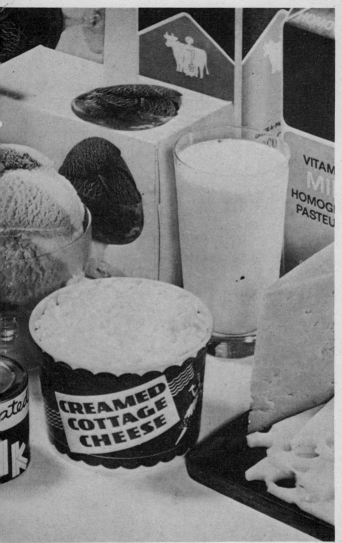

Choose with care.

Cereals
and Bread

The "Staff of Life," cereals and bread contain many of the B vitamins which contribute so greatly to our well-being.

You
May Eat:

Whole grain cereals
Unsweetened packaged cereals
Whole grain breads
Whole grain rolls
Brown rice
Barley
Dry, unsalted crackers
Enriched pasta (without heavy sauces)
Whole grain cookies

You May
Not Eat:

Sweetened packaged cereals
Salted nuts
Iced and frosted cakes
Pastries
**"Fake Foods" (potato, corn and
    other chips)**
White breads
Sweet rolls
Sweet breads

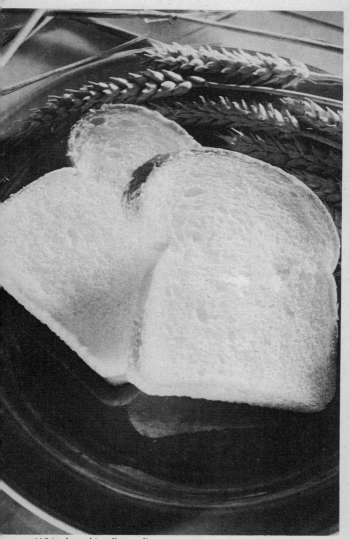

White bread is off your list.

Fruits and Vegetables

With vegetables, a good general rule is that anything you can eat raw — sliced, diced, shredded or
chopped into a salad — is a vegetable you can eat in
any amounts you can consume. The one notable
exception to the rule is the avocado. This delightful
food is almost too much of a good thing. True, it has
an incredible amount of vitamins and minerals
packed into its soft green flesh, but it has an equally
large number of calories as well, which keeps it off
many diets. A good compromise is, one-half an
avocado at a time. Eat it for lunch on a day when you
have company coming for dinner, and mash up the
remaining half with some oil and spices for gua-
camole, or avocado spread. And don't be so foolish
as to throw away the pit: An avocado pit, planted
rounded end down, turns into a marvelous indoor
tree.

You
May Eat:

All "salad" vegetables
(cabbage, lettuce,
radishes, onions,
mushrooms, zucchini,
tomatoes, celery,
white turnips,
carrots, green peas,
watercress, parsley,
cucumber, spinach,
potatoes)
Also: Boiled potatoes,
baked potatoes
Lentils, soybeans, dried peas*
Apples
Pears
Peaches
Melons
Grapes
Berries
Avocados (in limited
amounts)
Oranges
Grapefruits
Lemons**
Limes**
Ugli fruit
Guavas
Prunes and other dried
fruits

*Because these beans, or legumes, are an excellent source of
protein, they are generally considered part of the meat
group, rather than the fruit-vegetable, when planning a
daily diet.
**The juice of lemons and limes makes a marvelous, permis-
sible salad dressing when mixed with garlic and herbs.

You May Not Eat:

Canned vegetables (too much salt)
Fried vegetables
Canned fruits (too much sugar)
Olives*
Corn**
Pickles and sauerkraut†

*Olives have a high proportion of monounsaturated fats and are restricted on low-cholesterol diets.
**Corn is high in starch, but may be eaten in moderation.
†These are too high in salt and, although they are low in calories, may be irritating to the stomach on a diet.

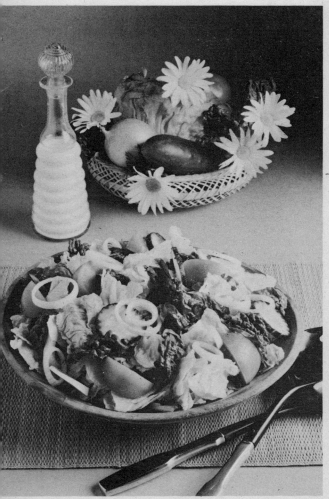

With a lemon juice dressing this salad would be perfect.

Liquids

You
May Drink:

Water
Decaffeinated "coffee"
Fruit and vegetable juices*
**Tisanes (teas brewed from
    various herbs, fruits
    and vegetables, steeped
    in boiling water, strained
    and served)**
**White wine (one glass only, on
    special occasions)**

*Fruit and vegetable juices should be regarded as liquids, not
as substitutes for fresh, raw vegetables and fruits which are
invaluable in helping the body eliminate wastes.

You May Not Drink:

Hard liquor
Carbonated beverages
Coffee
Hot chocolate
"Ades"
Bouillon brewed from cubes
   (This is to be avoided
   because of the excessive
   salt content. If you
   can find a salt-free
   version, by all means
   enjoy it. Otherwise
   make your own and enjoy
   it free of all unnecessary
   additives and polluting
   agents)

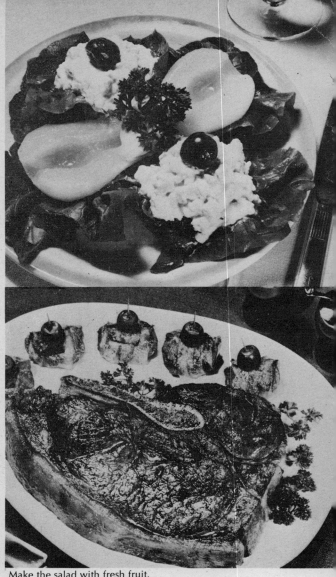

Make the salad with fresh fruit.

Don't eat beef more than three times a week.

How to Use This List

Because the Cellulite-control diet is a **cleansing,** rather than a reducing, diet, the foods on the list may be used in a variety of ways.

You may, for example, integrate them into your present diet. Or you may set up a rigidly controlled weekly meal and menu plan, following a caloric-reduction principle. (If you do this, however, be certain not to turn it into a starvation or fad diet. Remember, the Cellulite-control program demands that you not create additional stress for your body.) Finally, you may experiment, by creating a series of five, six or seven small meals which you will consume each day in place of the accustomed three large meals. Recent nutritional studies, in fact, have shown this last to be highly beneficial to the system.

The choice is yours. Just remember to stick to the

foods on the list; to be certain to include selections from each of the four major food groups in each day's plan; to consume the required amount of liquids; and, always, to check with your doctor before making any drastic changes in your normal dietary regime.

A Final Word About Nutrition: Vitamins

Despite the ease with which they are dispensed and purchased, vitamins are medicine and ought never to be casually prescribed. To emphasize this point, the Federal government has recently released material documenting the toxic effects of overdoses of vitamins A and D, and, as a result, has limited the amount of each vitamin which can be packed into a single pill.

If you really feel that you must have a vitamin to supplement your daily diet (although you should have quite enough vitamins by choosing carefully from each of the four food groups), you may pick one of the standard multi-vitamin prescriptions. By the way, the one exception to the rule is iron. Most women in this country really do not get enough iron in their daily diet, so they should include a multi-vitamin which has iron in it, or, if they prefer, a simple iron supplement alone.

As with diet, however, always check with your doctor before adding any supplement at all.

Exercise for Cellulite Control

Just as no proper diet should leave your body starved and stressed, no exercise intended to assist in Cellulite control should ever leave you weak and exhausted. Pleasantly tingly, yes; weak and trembly, never.

While you won't be able to avoid the inevitable muscle aches which come with the start of a new exercise regime, you should never make them worse by rushing into a strenuous schedule with little or no preparation. Take your time. Start with walking and build up to a mile or two or three a day. Add a few exercises for your problem areas, always a bit at a time. Start with say, 10 minutes of these problem-solvers and then work up to no more than 25 minutes a day. Remember, your aim is to assist your body in its attempt to rid itself of ugly Cellulite deposits — not to work yourself into an Olympic champion in two weeks flat.

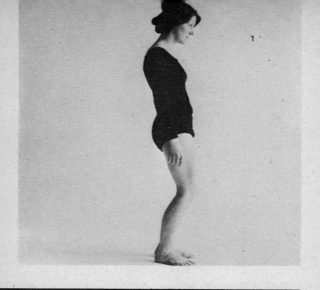

Breathing Right

As you know, proper breathing — bringing in enough oxygen to assist your body in ridding itself of pollutants and waste material — is essential to your Cellulite-control program. And proper breathing starts with proper posture.

(1) This is bad posture. The shoulders are slumped, creating a constricted space within the rib cage which keeps the lungs from expanding to their full capacity. In addition, the head is falling forward, creating a strain on the neck muscles. Altogether, a bad bargain.

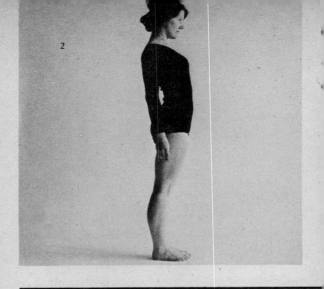

2

(2) This is also bad posture. Once the ideal of the legendary West Point cadets, this exaggerated and tense position constricts your muscles and can produce only strain and discomfort.

(3) This is the way good posture looks — relaxed and natural, with the body weight evenly distributed. There is no added strain on any one set of muscles, and the lungs are allowed full room for expansion within the chest.

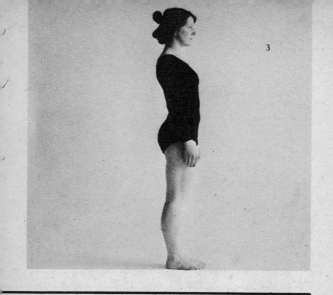

3

One more note on breathing: Nature provided an exceedingly efficient system for bringing air into the body, while warming and cleaning it at the same time. This system is simply breathing through the nose, which takes the air through a natural filter system of cilia (or small hairs) which remove most pollutants and warm the in-rushing breath. Although the sophisticated debris found in modern city air may often defeat even this system of the upper respiratory tract, breathing through the nose is still preferable in daily living. Breathing through the mouth should be used specifically to provide quick gulps of air in special exercising.

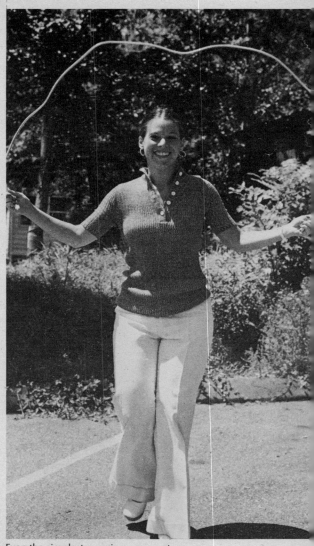

Even the simplest exercises are good.

Bringing Air in— Fast!

There are exercises which bring air in fast, and these are often used as warm-up exercises to start your daily session of Cellulite — control physical maintenance.

The first is an old childhood favorite, jumping rope. You can find a jump-rope at your neighborhood toy or candy store, and that's all the equipment you require. Just jump, and you'll be surprised at how much better you feel. Don't overdo it, though. As with all serious exercise programs, even so simple a thing as jumping rope should be taken slowly, until you have built up your stamina. Start with 10 jumps of the rope and build up to 50 by increasing the exercise 10 jumps per week.

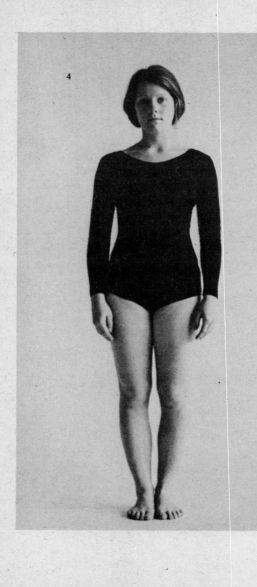

4

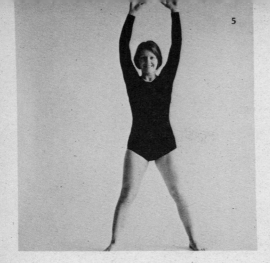

The second exercise to bring air in quickly is also an old favorite, one we call the "Jumping Jack."

Start, (4) with your hands at your sides and your feet together and jump (5) so that your hands are flung over your head and your feet are apart and then jump back to starting position. Repeat this three times in quick succession between exercises to build up your oxygen capacity.

All-over Athletics

Ordinary reducing diets often promote a schedule of various athletic pursuits in an effort to "burn off" calories. The aim of the Cellulite-control program, however, is to eliminate the unsightly, unevenly distributed lumps and bumps of fat which you find at vulnerable body points. As a result, the program specifically avoids such sports as tennis, horseback riding, or even ballet — pursuits which will defeat your Cellulite-control efforts by adding muscles bulges to your Cellulite bumps.

Instead, the Cellulite-control program recommends three specific "all-over" activities, activities which promote a smooth distribution of body fat and flesh, thus speeding you on your way to a newer, smoother body structure.

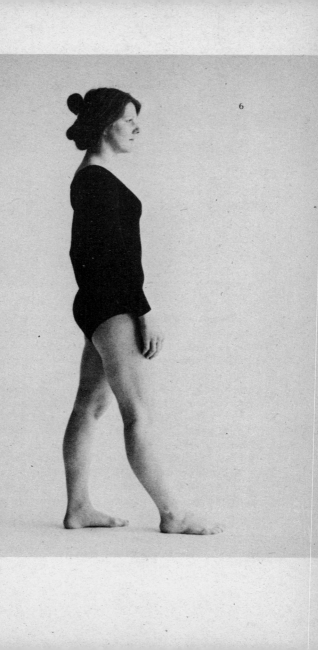

6

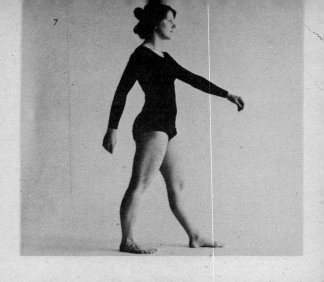

Perhaps the best of the "all-over" exercises is walking. That's right, just plain ordinary walking, one foot after the other. There is scarcely another athletic endeavor which uses the muscle structure of the body with such precision and economy. You begin (6) with proper posture, and, as you walk (7) your leg muscles swing forward, your torso muscles support your internal organs, your arms and shoulder muscles swing, your neck muscles support your head and even the muscles of your eyes work as your eyes watch where you are going.

In addition, walking has convenience to recommend it. Everybody has the opportunity to walk during every day, and would be better for taking advantage of the chance. To repeat, there is scarcely

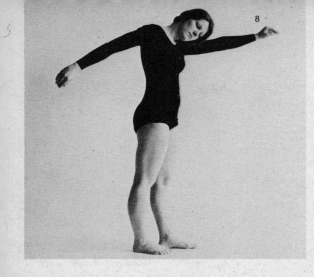

a better exercise to add to your Cellulite-control program.

Swimming is another "all-over" activity which uses all the muscles of your body to promote a smooth distribution of body flesh. If you can't make it to the beach or to a pool often enough, you can still use some of the muscle movements on dry land.

For example, (8) the arm movements of the Australian crawl, (9) provide an excellent opportunity to work Cellulite off the upper arms and back. This exercise is particularly good for women with flabby upper arms and men who are subject to the traditionally male placement of Cellulite on the upper back.

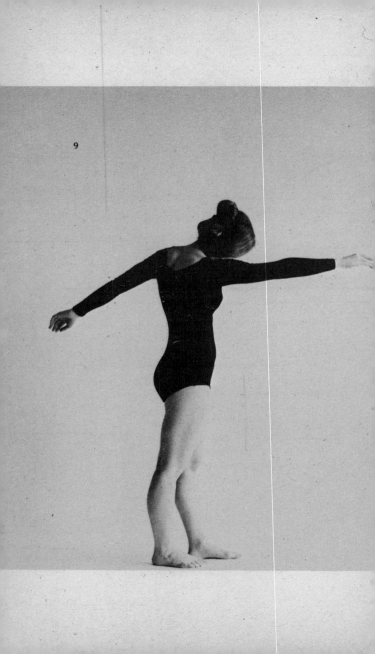

9

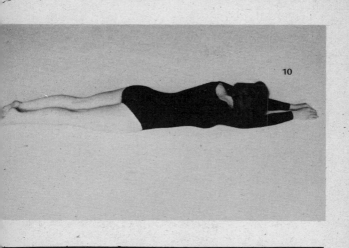

Then, too, you can benefit from the "all-over" effect of swimming, even in your own living room, with this muscle worker: (10) lie flat on the floor in the "dead man's float" position. Then, (11) lift your arms and legs from the ground. This is a difficult exercise at first and the position should not be held longer than the count of 1-2. Once you get the hang of it, however, you will feel its benefits all over your body.

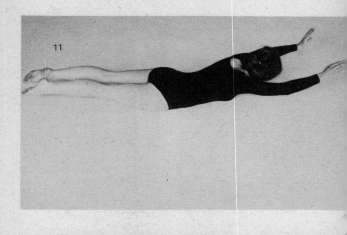

11

Finally, that old favorite, modern dance, is an excellent part of your Cellulite-control program. Modern dance's benefit lies in the fact that it stretches many of our muscles at once, thereby providing a smoother effect which is missing in the more rigidly structured ballet. Reach (12), bend, stretch, and generally work away your Cellulite. If you prefer, you should do this to the tune of your favorite records. And as a matter of fact, music, with its natural rhythms, is an excellent accompaniment to any exercise schedule. You will find that it relaxes you, provides a "beat" to work to, and generally makes the exercise time whizz by.

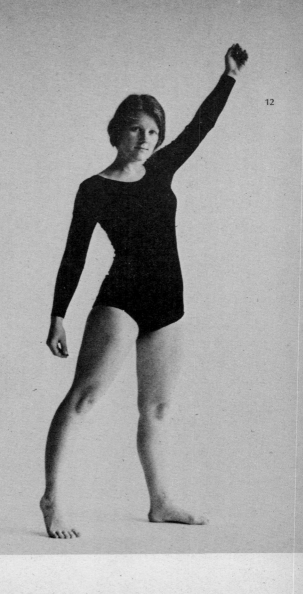

12

Special Exercises for Special Effects

The Upper Arms

Cellulite on the upper arms is usually a condition afflicting older women or women who have been seriously obese. The following exercises are designed to tighten up these areas and eliminate the flabby Cellulite deposits. (In addition, these exercises are fine for men whose Cellulite deposits are settled into clumps on the upper back.)

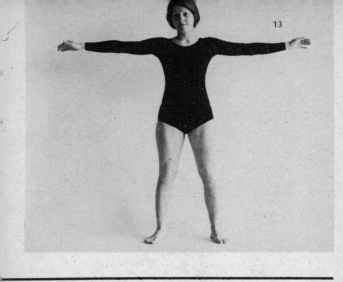

13

Start with arms out (13) and then rotate arms backward in circles (14). You should begin with small circles in which the arms rotate approximately four inches, and then proceed to build up the circles until you are swinging your arms in great circles which stretch over your head and almost to your waist. Take it slowly, though, or you will have unnecessary muscle strain.

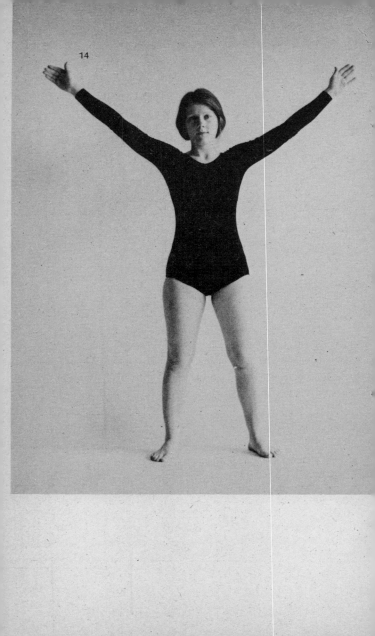
14

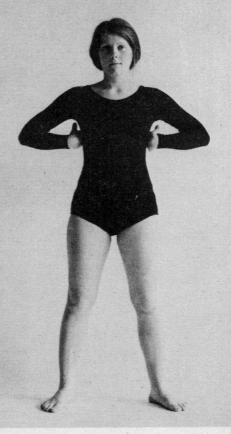

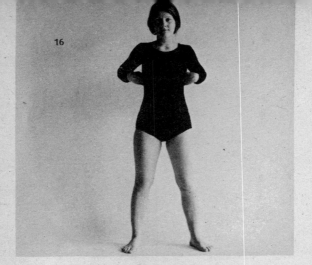

16

A second exercise for this problem area is called "The Chicken." Start (15) with your arms tucked up into "wings" at your sides and then (16), pull your elbows back. As you do so, you will feel the muscles in your upper arms and back responding.

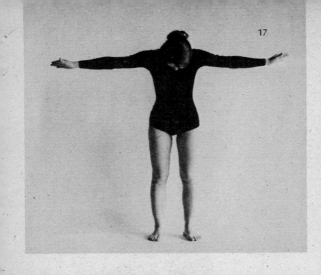

Your upper arms and back will also respond to this "Arm Cross Swing." Start with your arms out (17) and your head down. Then swing your arms down and cross them (18). Finish by swinging your arms back to starting position. **NOTE:** Always keep your head down while doing this exercise.

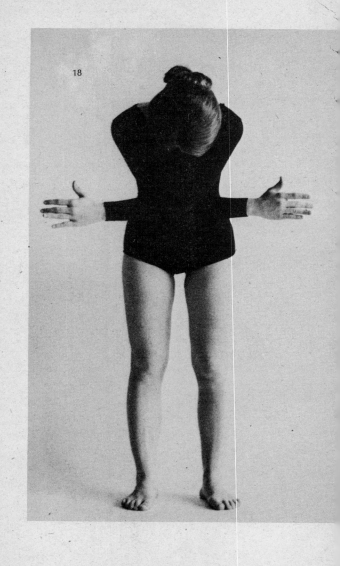

The Midriff

Cellulite bulges around the midriff and waist can be a special trial in today's clinging clothes, not to mention the fact that they make it impossible to wear a two-piece or bikini bathing suit. Fortunately, these ugly bumps respond rather quickly to a series of classic twisting exercises.

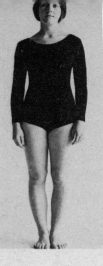

19

The sequence begins with the standard starting position (19). Then, bend to one side, stretching your arm down as far as you can reach while keeping your feet flat on the floor and your knees straight. Bend to one side (20). Return to the starting position, and switch the exercise to the other side. Repeat five times on each side.

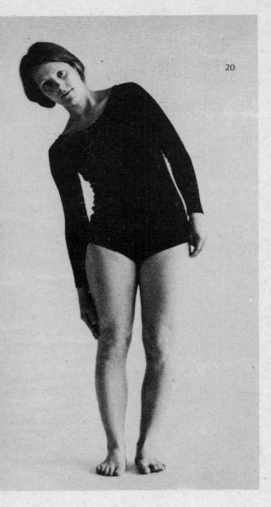

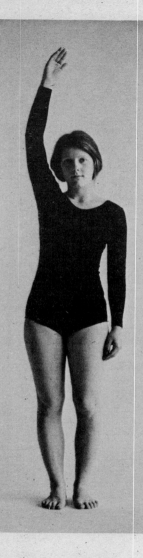

21

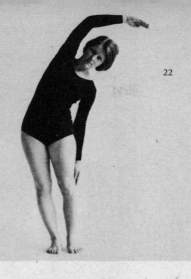

22

As your muscles and bulges begin to respond, you can go on to the next exercise in the series. Begin (21), with one arm over your head, then (22) bend so that the arm arcs over your head. Return to starting position, with other arm over head and switch to the other side. Repeat the exercise five times on each side.

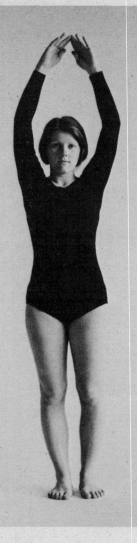

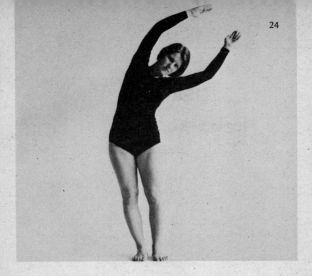

24

Finally, you will progress to the most strenuous of
the series. Begin (23) with both arms over your head.
Then (24) stretch to one side. Return to starting position and stretch to the other side. Repeat five times
on each side.

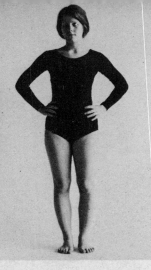

25

Another twist exercise of use in whittling down your midriff and waist is this. Start (25) with both arms on your hips. Then (26) twist to the side. Return to starting position, and twist to other side. Repeat five times to each side.

You should begin to see the effects of these exercises within the second week, as you move on to the second of the stretching exercises. You can, of course, switch back and forth at will among these four exercises.

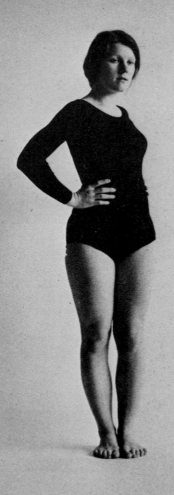

Hips and buttocks

Working down the body, you will come to Cellulite bulges on the hips and buttocks, a particular problem for women afflicted with the Cellulite scourge. Attack the problem areas with these exercises.

Start by sitting on the floor (27), then "walk" backwards on your buttocks. After 10 "steps," reverse the process and "walk" forward 10 "steps."

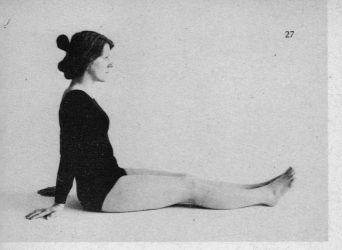

27

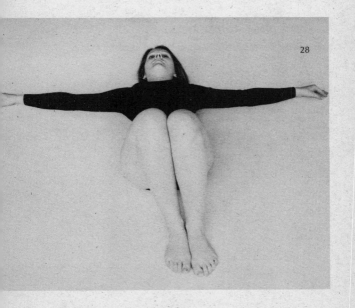

28

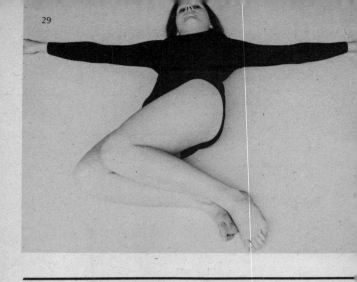

This will work to whittle your waist as well as your hips and buttocks. Start by lying on the floor (28) with your knees bent. Then, twist knees to one side (29). Return to starting position and twist to other side. Repeat five times on each side.

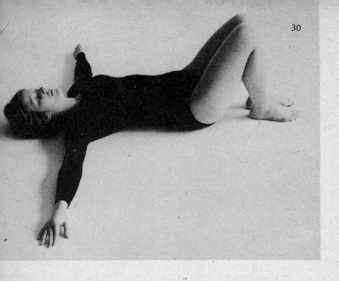

The position for the classic bicycle exercise often demands that the hips be raised into the air and the entire body be supported by the back and shoulders. This position, however, is quite strenuous and, if done wrong, can sometimes result in seriously strained muscles. The position shown here (30) is a less strained one from which to begin. Lie on the floor with your knees bent. Then, (31) lift your legs and (32) just bicycle away. This will necessarily restrict your motions, but it will provide all the benefits of the more strenuous position with none of the drawbacks.

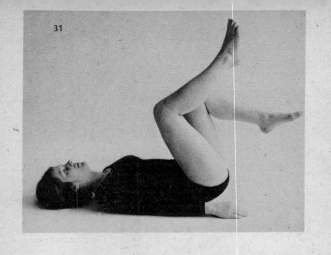

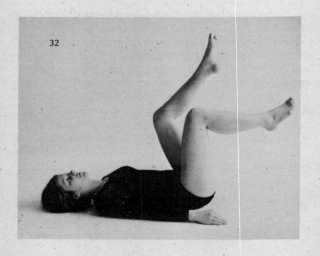

The
Thighs

Exercises designed to get after the classic **coulottes de cheval** ("riding breechs," or Cellulite deposits on the upper thigh) have the delightful side
effect of working to eliminate Cellulite on the hips
and buttocks as well. So intimately are these trouble
areas connected, that each of the following will
yield you multiple dividends in your fight to do
away with Cellulite bulges and bumps.

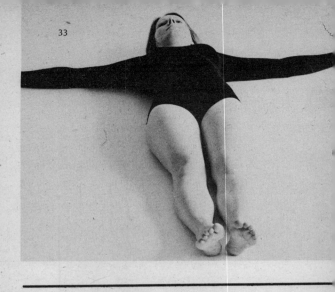

33

To stretch and smooth the upper thigh, start (33) lying flat on the floor, with arms outstretched and legs together. Then (34) lift and cross one leg over the other. Return to starting position, and switch to the other side (35). As you progress, try to lift the leg higher and higher as you cross over, so that your ideal is to touch the leg to the opposite hand. Don't strain, however; this ultimate ideal is **very** difficult to achieve.

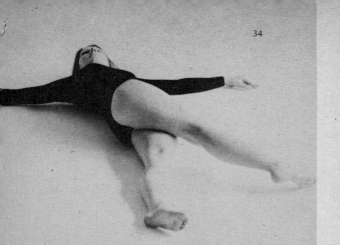

34

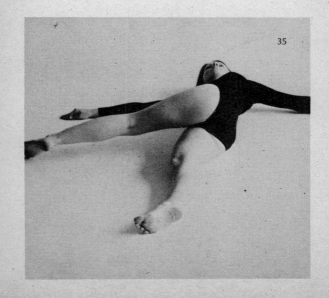

35

Another thigh smoother with multiple benefits is this. Kneel on the floor (36) and bring your knee up to your nose. Then, **smoothly** stretch out the leg (37). Repeat on the other side. The key to this exercise is to do it smoothly. Never, never kick your leg out abruptly, lest you injure a back muscle in the process.

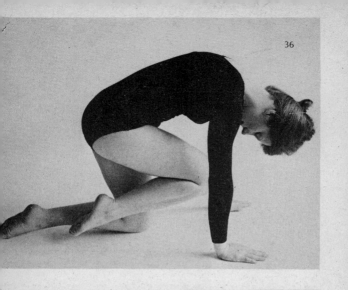

36

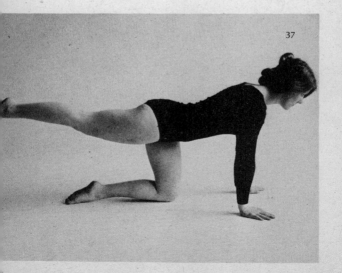

37

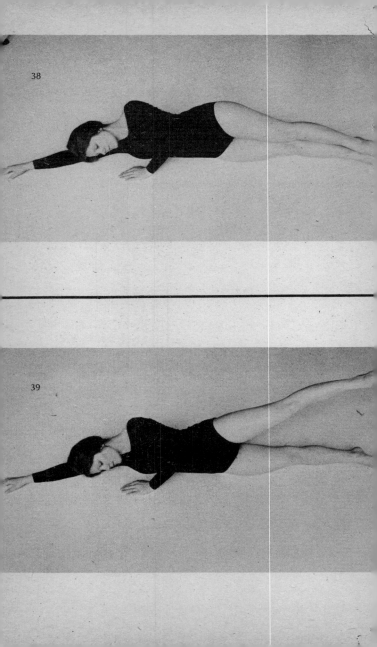

A final stretcher for the upper thigh is this one. Lie on your side (38), supporting yourself with your arms. Then lift your leg (39) and hold it aloft for the count of three. Lower the leg, repeat the exercise four times, then switch to the other side.

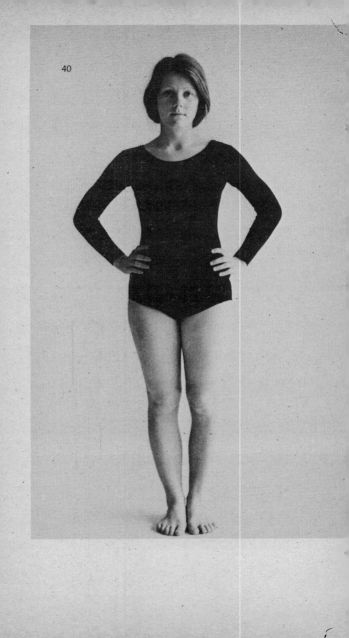

40

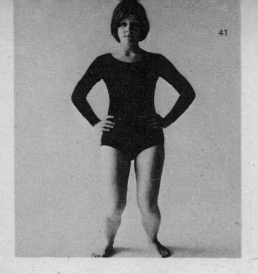

41

Finally, the classic deep-knee bend is great for smoothing out the upper thigh. Start (40) with hands on hips, and then, (41) bend. It's that simple. And it works.

Massage
Techniques

Massage assists your body to eliminate Cellulite deposits by toning up the circulation in specific areas. In addition, it leaves you with a delightful tingling, yet relaxed sensation which is hard to beat in any program of physical maintenance.

You start your self-massage program with a simple finger-tip touch. It's shown here on the upper thigh (42) where Cellulite is most likely to clump.

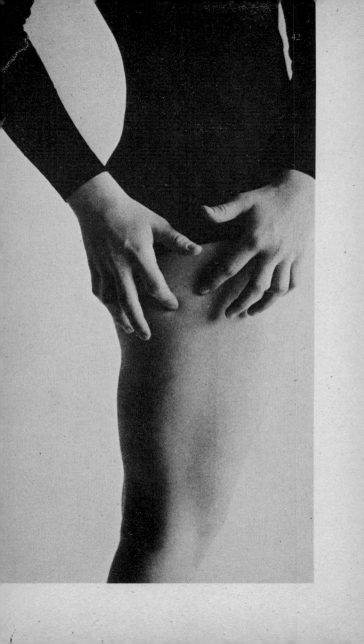

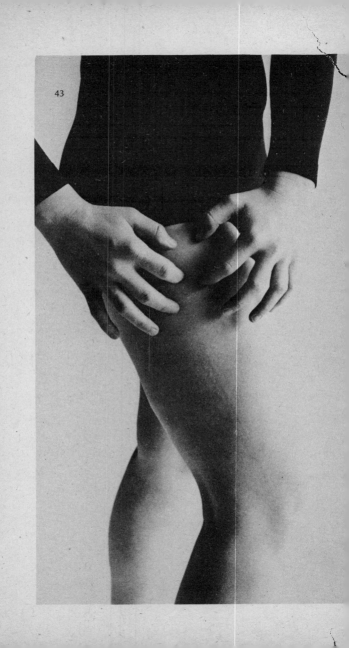

43

You can increase the pressure of the finger tips (43), to produce a deeper impression, but under no condition should you ever leave bruises on the skin.

Your palm is another instrument of massage (44). Begin by pressing the palm into the Cellulite deposit, then (45) rotate the palm in a circle pattern. Repeat 10 times.

The two-hand twist is a third effective method of self-massage. Gently (46) take the Cellulite into your hands, and then, again, gently (47) twist in opposite directions. You may increase the pressure, but **never** to the point of actual pain.

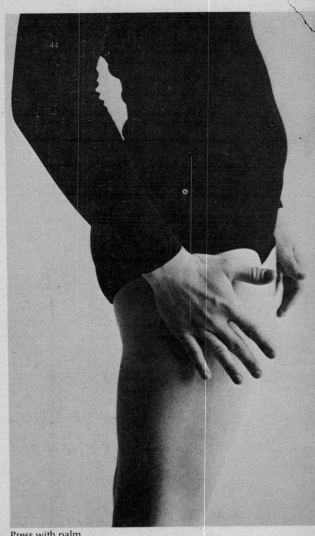

Press with palm . . .

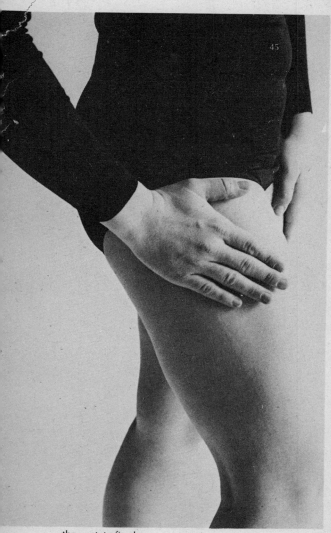

45

... then rotate firmly.

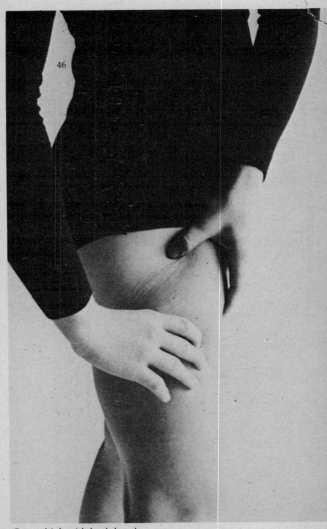

46

Grasp thigh with both hands.

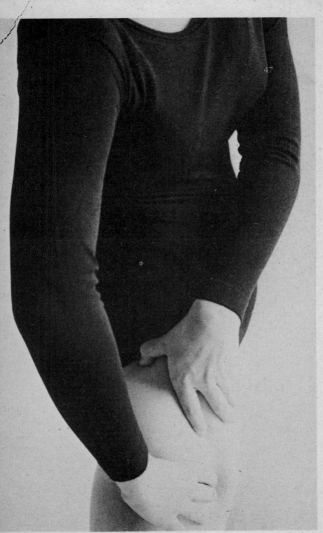

Then twist *gently* in opposite directions.

A dry towel is also a great way to massage yourself. Use it on the upper back (48), on the buttocks (49), or on the upper thigh (50). Always hold the towel tightly in your hands and rub it briskly over the skin surface. This will leave you feeling absolutely tip-top, tingly and deliciously stimulated.

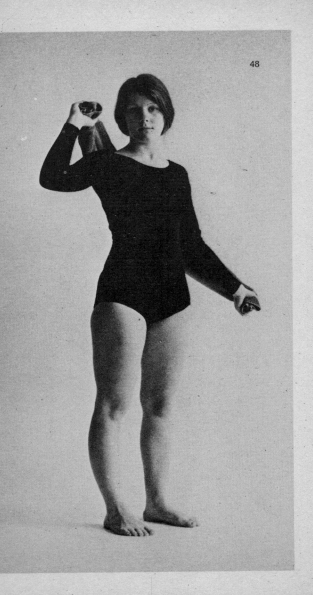

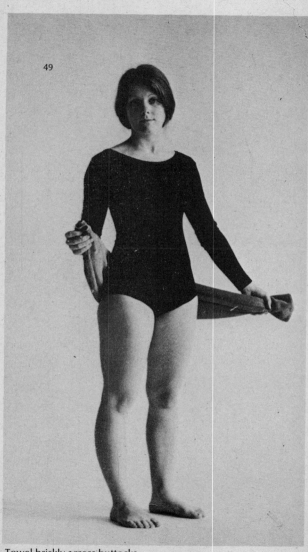

49

Towel briskly across buttocks . . .

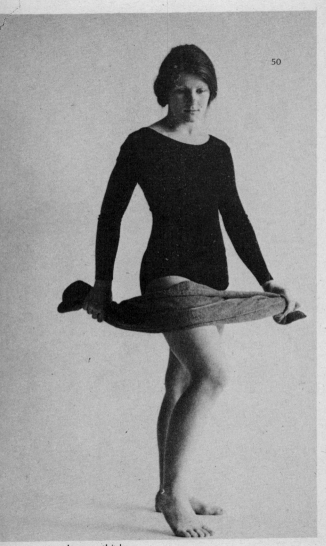

. . . and upper thighs.

The **loofa,** a Swedish sponge or mitt, is another instrument of massage. The **loofa** belongs in your bath and should be used (51) wet, while you are showering. Like the dry towel massage, this will smooth your skin, flaking off the dry outer layer and leaving you smooth as the proverbial baby.

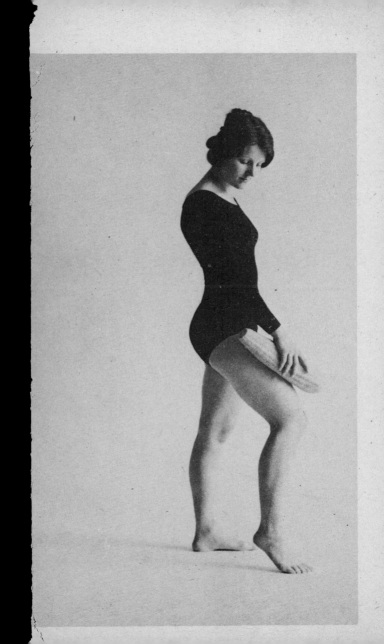

Afterword

As you have seen, the Cellulite-control program is sensible, safe, easy to follow. It involves no drugs, no starvation or fad diets, no Olympic training. You can, if you think about it, plan for yourself a program of diet and exercise which fits right in with your everyday way of life (and don't forget to check with your doctor before doing anything drastically different). Experiment a little with the choices given. There are enough of them to suit a wide range of life styles.

The road to Cellulite-control is not to be thought of as a race track. You must begin your journey slowly and carefully. Take the time to plan out your Cellulite-control menus (your family has to live with them too), and to learn to perform the massages and exercises for their maximum benefit to you. It will be time well spent, for it will allow you greater speed later on. You will find that the Cellulite-control program has become second nature, so that you can easily follow it your whole life long.

And always remember that it is **your** life and **your** body you are working for. Never become trapped in a race against next season's fashions, or a contest with the dieter next door. As the saying goes, "haste makes waste," — and "waste" is exactly what you are working to eliminate from your body. So, take it easy with yourself. Keep your food intake satisfying and varied — there are plenty of permissible foods from which to choose. Build up gradually to the suggested numbers of exercises. Don't ever massage yourself black and blue — a properly performed massage should leave you feeling wonderful. Above all, bear in mind that the most important lesson of this book is to try to avoid shocking or straining your body. The key word in Cellulite-control is "moderation."

Of all the bodies Nature designed, mankind was given the best. **You** are the strongest living creature on earth. You have a body which can adapt itself to all the different conditions of life on this planet. You owe it to yourself to keep that body running at top form, smoothly, free of choking wastes. With a little determination, and the guidelines you have learned from this book, you can do so. You will feel like the marvelous being you are, as you enjoy the full potential of the Cellulite-free you. And you will look (as those wise Frenchmen put it) "Magnifique!"

Selected Bibliographical Sources

Cellulite

The first American magazine to publish information about Cellulite was *Vogue,* which ran "Cellulite" in its April 15, 1968 issue. *Vogue* also discussed Cellulite in the "Beauty Bulletin" (November 1, 1970), "The Beauty Checkout" (May, 1973) and in numerous other articles.

In January, February and March, 1971, *Harper's Bazaar* ran a series of interviews with Cellulite-expert Nicole Ronsard (who is, in turn, author of *Cellulite,* New York: Beauty and Health Press).

For the European view, see Princess Luciana Pignatelli's *The Beautiful People's Beauty Book* (New York: Bantam Books) which describes some of the treatments available on the Continent.

Nutrition and Diet

Glenn, Morton, M.D. *How to Get Thinner Once and For All*. Greenwich, Connecticut: Fawcett Publications.

221

Gwinup, Grant, M.D. *Energetics*. Los Angeles: Sherbourne Press, Inc.

Margolius, Sidney. *Health Foods, Facts and Fakes*. New York: Walker & Company.

Nidetch, Jean. *The Story of Weight Watchers*. New York: Signet Books.

Solomon, Neil, M.D. *The Truth About Weight Control*. New York: Dell Publishing Co., Inc.

Ubell, Earl. *How to Save Your Life*. New York: Harcourt, Brace, Jovanovich, Inc.

Williams, Roger. *Nutrition Against Disease*. New York: Pitman Publishing Corp.

Entertaining essays on general health

Eckstein, Gustav. *The Body Has a Head*. New York: Harper and Row, Publishers, Inc.

Lang, Theo. *The Difference Between a Man and a Woman*. New York: The John Day Company, Inc.

Rosebury, Theodore. *Life On Man*. New York: Berkeley Publishing Corp.

Exercise

Ald, Roy. *Jump For Joy*. New York: Bernard Geis Associates, Inc.

Goode, Ruth and Sussman, Aaron. *The Magic of Walking*. New York: Simon and Schuster.

The Israel Army Physical Fitness Book. New York: Grosset & Dunlap, Inc.

Prudden, Bonnie. *How to Keep Slender and Fit After Thirty*. New York: Pocket Books.

Cookbooks

Bennett, Iva and Simon, Martha. *The Prudent Diet*. New York: Bantam Books.

Fisher, M.F.K. *The Art of Eating*. New York: Macmillan, Inc.

Rombauer, Irma S. and Becker, Marion Rombauer. *The Joy of Cooking*. Indianapolis: The Bobbs-Merrill Co., Inc.

PHOTO CREDITS

The editors gratefully acknowledge the cooperation of the following agencies and organizations in providing photographs for use in this book.